IKIGAI

GAETANO FORTUGNO

TABLE OF CONTENTS

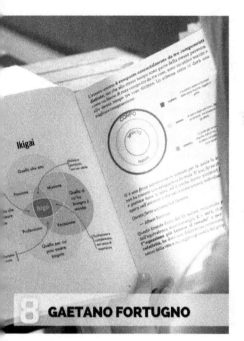

8 GAETANO FORTUGNO

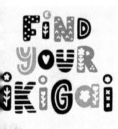

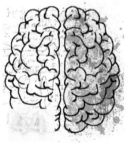

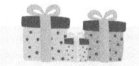

TABLE OF CONTENTS

A challenge for you

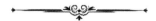

You will understand later. Take paper and pencil and draw 9 points like this:

1. **MAXIMUM TRACK 4 LINES**
2. **TAP ALL POINTS**
3. **WITHOUT EVER DETACHING THE PENCIL FROM THE SHEET**

You can try as many times as you want.

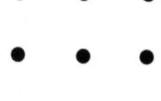

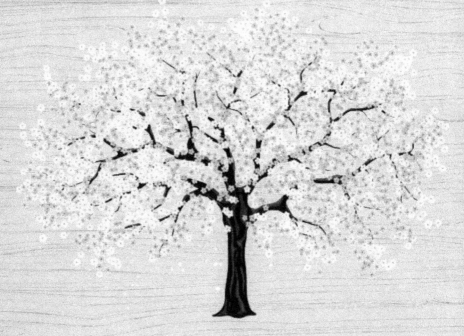

GRAB WISDOM, DON'T SELL IT

SENSE, FOR THOSE WHO POSSESS IT, IS A SOURCE OF LIFE, BUT FOOLISHNESS IS THE PUNISHMENT OF FOOLS.

Who is it Gaetano Fortugno

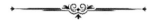

Gaetano Fortugno is an Italian writer, always been attracted by spirituality. Born in Italy in 1980 to Italian parents, he has a strong sensitivity and a propensity to seek the purpose of life. He begins his inner journey in search of concrete answers to the great questions of human existence.

About us? Why do we live? What is the meaning of life?

Examining the great contradiction between the professed creed and the daily reality of the great religions, he decides to experience firsthand what offers concrete feedback. He refuses to have theoretical, notional knowledge and is not followed by real-life experiences.

The author goes through periods of crisis, followed by a spiritual awakening. This very intense phase is conducted along a path made of compelling practical experiences.

It lives part of its existence in poor conditions, economically and materially. Thanks to his strong determination and tenacity, he manages to find the purpose of his life, to become free and live a whole and joyful existence.

Letter to my readers

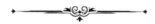

entile reader, thank you for choosing this humble literary work. I hope I have succeeded in conveying my message clearly and concisely. Forgive any possible imperfections; I have personally sketched and corrected this manual to offer unfiltered content as close as possible to my experiences. Consider it as a handicraft, beautiful precisely because of its imperfection. I intend to provide a quality text that maintains a solid social utility.

If you are attentive and read with pure sincerity, it will help you receive a new life by discovering your *ikigai*. The guide will show you how to leave the hectic life behind, helping you find your purpose, to live a whole life.

Japanese believe that everyone has an *ikigai,* so we jump out of bed every morning.

I hope you read this book as a child would, free from all prejudice and with the desire to surprise you. This book will only be a book for some people, but it will substantially impact others. This treatise will lead you along the path of my personal experiences. It will look like turning on a light. Light can produce two different reactions, or it will bother the eyes, or it will be welcomed to be illuminated. I do not think I can lead you to this experience with my forces, I will limit myself to being a road sign to show you the direction, but the road will be you to travel it. In any case, the signal remains only a signal; it is the crucial goal.

Children simply reason great mysteries. Si expresses without the filter of prejudices; they reveal hidden things. Have you ever watched a child look at a butterfly? Can you get excited about a butterfly or a bird-like the little ones do? Let's start taking them as an example. You have to become like little children.

I also want to tell you that this book is not a classic manual that will tell you exactly what to do, limiting itself to giving you notions, but I will let the concepts that inspired me and gave me results come out spontaneously from these pages. You will be the one to grasp the nuances and lessons that you can assimilate, also based on your degree of sensitivity.

Ikigai etymology

The words have a profound meaning in Giappone; they reflect a lifestyle that is difficult to understand. Ikigai alike; translating it into two or three words would be insufficient.

Iki is a Japanese term meaning "existence" or "life." Gai is a Greek word meaning "reason" or "purpose." Translation has to do with "purpose of life" or "reason to exist."

This definition is the most accurate translation. The message, however, is much more profound. Ikigai is the invisible force that pushes you out of bed every morning.

It is the reason that makes it worth facing the outside world, with all its challenges. IKIGAI is the realization of our innermost desires, ambitions, and vocations.

In the end, it is to find our reason for existing so that we do not remain an invisible dot in the universe; it is our brief presence on this planet that leaves an indelible mark.

This book was written almost for a case; I have accumulated spiritual and material experiences that have allowed me to understand many realities over the years. I wanted to create something of real value that was unique and allowed me to leave my mark on this world. At the same time, I liked the experiences told to reflect my everyday reality. If you have asked yourself questions similar to the following, you are looking for something profound and not reading by chance.

What is the meaning of my life?

The point is to live longer, or should I seek a higher purpose? Few people find the authentic way and live with passion, while others languish in confusion. Have you wondered why?

The purpose of life may be a way to explain why the Japanese live so long, especially on the island of Okinawa, where there are 24.55 people over the age of 100 for every 100,000 people; this is a lot more than the global average.

Researchers are trying to figure out why people on this island in southern Japan live longer than anyone else. They think that a healthy diet, simple outdoor living, green tea, and a subtropical climate (the average temperature is about the same as Hawaii) are some of the factors. The ikigai, which shapes their lives, is one of them.

Is it the reason why there are more centenarians in Okinawa than elsewhere? How does it inspire people to stay active until the end? What is the secret to a long and happy life?

Ogimi is a rural town located in Kunigami District of Okinawa Prefecture. It has a population of about three thousand inhabitants. The village benefits from fertile soil; activities such as agriculture, breeding, fishing, and collecting certain types of algae are the main activities of the place. The crafts and ceramics of Ogimi are another foundation of the local economy.

Okinawa is where most of the *"shikuwasa"* is a lime-like fruit that encloses an extraordinary power antioxidant. **Could this be the secret? Or is it the purity of the water used to make Moringa tea?** In Ogimi, we talk an ancient dialect; the population is exceptionally kind and possesses a fantastic friendliness.

A group of scholars has interviewed some elderly residents in the past. After all, scholars realized something much more potent than these natural resources was at work: a unique joy flowed from its inhabitants. This inner joy guides them through the long and pleasant journey of their lives.

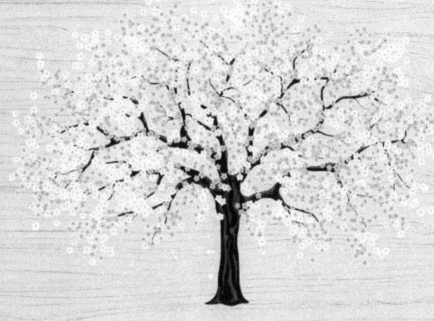

TRUE WISDOM IS LIFE

IT IS A TREE OF LIFE TO THOSE WHO TAKE IT,
AND WHOEVER POSSESSES IT IS BLESSED

Ikigai, what is it exactly? How do you get it?

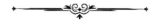

This lovely place arouses surprise in those who visit it; it seems impossible to conceive that two hundred thousand lives were lost in such a wonderful place during World War II. Rather than lock yourself up and nourish resentment towards the Foreign, the inhabitants of Okinawa live by the principle of *ichariba chode* ((行逢りば兄弟)), a local expression meaning "although we meet once, even by chance, We friends for life." Uno of the secrets of the happiness of the residents of Ogimi is taking care of others.

According to the old expression "Happier, what is giving than receiving," whoever gives something receives a joy that cannot be bought in any other way.

Caring for others, eating lightly, caring for the needs of the spirit, getting enough rest, taking joy in the little things in life, and exercising are habits that this group of people practices constantly.

Chi discovers his *ikigai has* everything he needs for a long and joyful journey in life.

Good reading!

What is the purpose of your existence?

Our lives gain peace, happiness, and purpose when we have a clear sense of our ikigai.

Ikigai

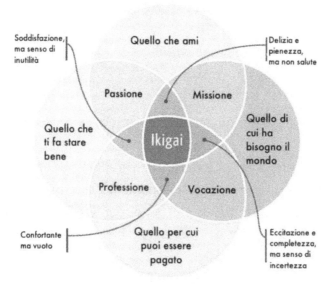

When you live in Japan, you'll notice how active retirees still are. Japanese many do not stop working.

According to National Geographic writer Dan Buettner, an expert on Japanese culture, "leave your job forever" does not exist in Japanese.

The ikigai asks you four questions to find out your reason for living

1. What is your favorite pastime?
2. What are your unique skills?
3. How can you contribute to the world?
4. You can be paid for what you do.

Finding answers to these questions and others can help us partially discover our true calling. One important thing is not to be in a hurry; for the Japanese, the Ikigai process is quite gradual and often has little to do with work or profits. Indeed, Ikigai leads to a better existence since it gives us a purpose to live and get out of bed every morning.

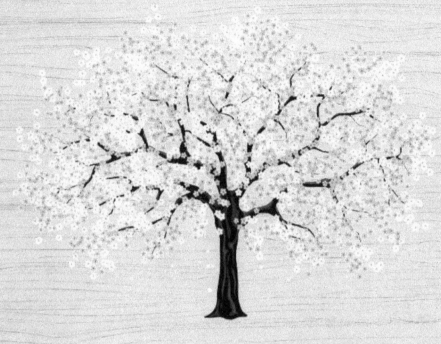

HOW TO NOURISH THE BODY

LIFE IS MORE THAN NOURISHMENT AND THE BODY MORE THAN CLOTHI

The Japanese diet

$\mathcal{T}$he Japanese diet is naturally high in nutrients, and beneficial compounds for health, including fiber, calcium, potassium, magnesium, iron, and vitamins A, C, and E. Vegetables contribute to the diet's nutritional richness and are frequently prepared in dashi, a broth of fish and marinated vegetables. This causes them to shrink in volume while increasing taste and digestibility, making it easier to consume large amounts.

There are also many algae and green tea in the diet. Foods are rich in antioxidants, natural substances that protect the body from cellular damage and disease. In addition, the diet's many fish and seaweed meals offer long-chain omega-three fats, which improve brain, eye, and heart health, and consume grains and legumes such as rice, soy, and quinoa. One study found that those who regularly practiced the traditional Japanese diet had a 15 percent reduced risk of premature mortality compared to those who did not.

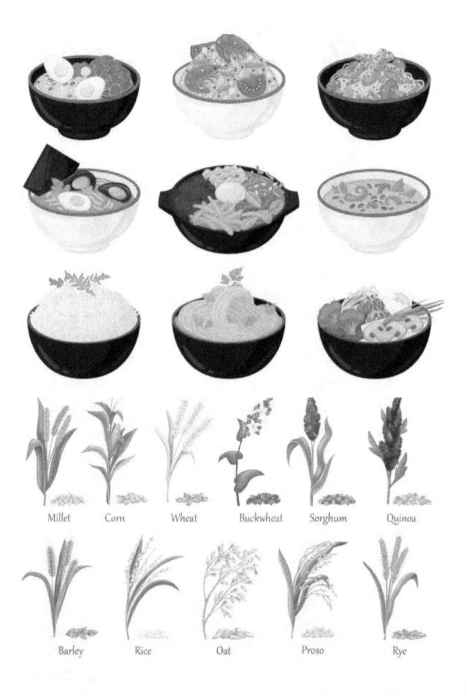

Millet   Corn   Wheat   Buckwheat   Sorghum   Quinoa

Barley   Rice   Oat   Proso   Rye

The 80% secret

One of the most common sayings in Japan is "**Hara Hachi bu,**" which is repeated before or after eating and means something like "Fill your belly to 80 percent". Okinawans stop eating when their stomach reaches 80% capacity, rather than overeating and wearing down their bodies with long digestive processes that accelerate cellular oxidation.

There's no way to know if your stomach is at 80% capacity, but the lesson to be learned from this saying is that we should stop eating when we start feeling full.

It's not just about what they eat, but also how they consume. Because their food is served on four small plates and one large one, the Japanese tend to eat less.

"HARA HACHI BU"

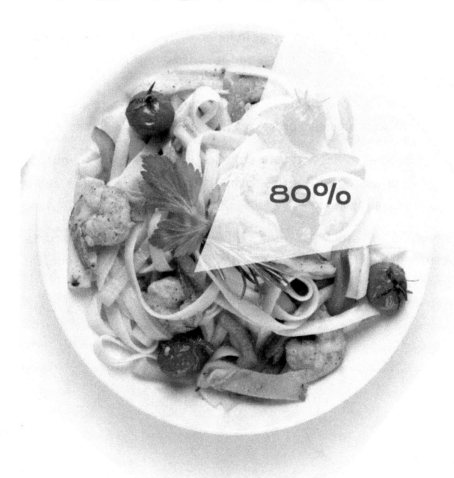

80%

You eat with your mouth and also with your mind, on a psychological level seeing more courses and full dishes helps you feel full.

Maintaining a young body

Yoshinori Ōsumi is a Japanese biologist who received the Nobel Prize in Medicine, thanks to a recent discovery concerning a physiological mechanism fundamental for cells' survival and the performance of their functions. Our cells constantly monitor their nutritional balance to conserve energy. Our cells continuously monitor their healthy balance to save energy. Caloric restriction such as fasting triggers natural mechanisms that promote cell turnover. This process increases the body's resistance to stress and helps its longevity. The human body has its **metabolism,** defined as synthetic biochemical reactions. The body can trigger two distinct phases; it can be found in the anabolic or catabolic phase.

- **Anabolism** (derived **from the Greek ἀναβάλλειν** is equivalent to **"pull up or build)** is the process of cell synthesis to create new living organic material within the body; this process requires energy, usually provided by food.

- **Catabolism (which** comes **from the Greek.** *katabállō* 'jet **down**) is the body's chemical process that uses "dismantling" organic material to produce energy; it is defined as a downward process in a sense like a bricklayer knocking down a wall. The fuel needed to produce energy is obtained primarily using organic material derived from digestion, and in the absence of resources, it uses part of the biological tissue.

Autophagy or auto-phagocytosis is the name of the mechanism discovered by Yoshinori. It is a word composed of auto- (from the Greek α ὑτός meaning "same") and -pheasant from the slang φαγεῖν, i.e., "to eat." Autophagy, therefore, signs "eating oneself"—the process of renewal of the cells that represent the building blocks of our body.

They were balancing opportunely, anabolism and catabolism, especially practicing controlled fasting. Healthy cells engulf old, worn, weak cells and convert them into energy. This function allows a cell turnover causing a kind of rejuvenation.

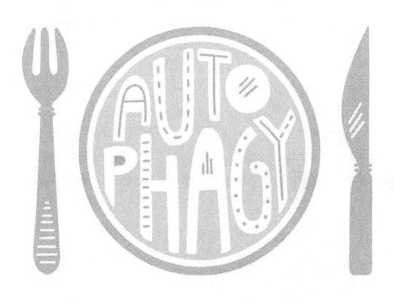

Autophagy Stages

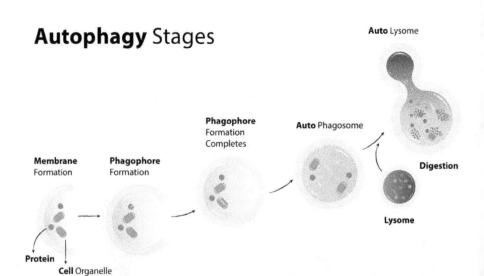

Auto Lysome

Phagophore
Formation
Completes

Auto Phagosome

Membrane
Formation

Phagophore
Formation

Digestion

Protein

Cell Organelle

Lysome

Scholars (such as the doctors of the Umberto Veronesi foundation) claim that dysfunctions in the mechanism of autophagy are implicated in many diseases, including **Parkinson's disease, diabetes, cancer, and many immune system disorders.** Autophagy is necessary for an individual's life; it copes with stressful conditions, such as malnutrition. **An adult needs about 250 grams of protein** daily. Digestion, on average, stores less protein than necessary; this means that a portion of protein is made up of cell recycling. Autophagy is also essential for eliminating external aggressors such as viruses, bacteria, and intracellular germs.

Obstacles to sleep

Abraham Haim of the University of Haifa researched the consequences of exposure to blue light produced by white LED lights and LED screens. Abraham has shown that exposure to this shade can decrease melatonin production.

The blue light acts directly on melanopsin, a protein found in some sensitive cells. These cells, in turn, affect our brain with adverse effects on the sleep-wake cycle.

The frequencies have the most significant effect between 440 and 460 nm. White LEDs emit blue light at 450 nm.

The circadian rhythm is vital, as its disruption can lead to conditions ranging from obesity to cancer.

SLEEP CYCLE

STAGE 1
light sleep & can be
easily awakened

STAGE 2
eye movement
& brain waves
slowing down

STAGE 3
delta waves begin
to appear

STAGE 4
deep sleep,
difficult to wake up

REM STAGE
breathing becomes
more rapid
& irregular

To avoid severe scenarios, experts advise informing consumers about the wavelength of light by affixing a label on the LED light box.

In addition, you should not use screen devices before sleeping.

Several essential processes occur during sleep. Many nocturnal functions promote brain health and overall fitness, especially in children and adolescents.

Brain and sleep

Not getting enough rest creates difficulties in making decisions, solving problems, experiencing emotions, and adapting to change. Sleep also plays an essential role in memory consolidation and selecting information received daily.

Sleeping has positive effects on the mechanism of removal of toxins accumulated by the brain. One of these toxins is beta-amyloid, a protein linked to Alzheimer's. The glymphatic system, so named for its resemblance to the lymphatic system, allows cerebrospinal fluid to move through the brain channels during sleep.

A good sleep cycle also helps regulate hormones such as ghrelin and leptin, which govern appetite and satiety, explaining the relationship between rest and obesity. Some hormones such as insulin, which regulates blood sugar, can alter, increasing blood sugar. Chronic sleep deprivation increases the risk of heart disease, stroke, diabetes, and kidney disease.

Night rest is closely linked to the processes of growth and development. Stimulates the production of hormones that increase muscle mass and repair cells and tissues.

Finally, the quality of rest is an indicator of daytime productivity at work or school. People who don't sleep spend more time completing tasks, make more mistakes, and have slower response times.

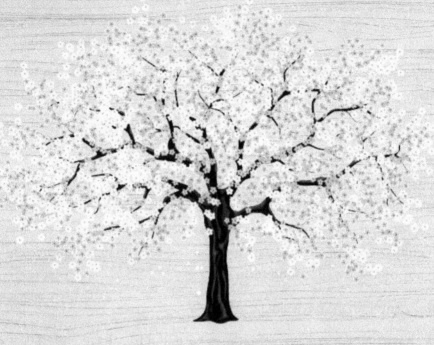

KEEP AN ACTIVE MIND

IN THE OLD YOU WILL FIND WISDOM

Coping with aging

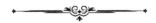

Many doctors believe that keeping the body young keeps the mind active.

> - **An essential component of ikigai is not to give up when we encounter difficulties.**

According to research conducted at Yeshiva University, individuals who live longer have two characteristics: a cheerful attitude and a high level of emotional awareness. In other words, individuals who face difficulties with a good mood and can control their emotions are already on their way to long-term success.

Many centenarians have similar profiles:

They have had entire lives, sometimes hard, but they have understood how to face these difficulties with a good attitude so as not to be overwhelmed by the barriers they have encountered.

Alexander Imich, who became the oldest man in the world at the age of 111 in 2014, knew he had good genes but also realized that other factors played a role:

"The quality of life you live is important for longevity," he said in an interview with Reuters after being listed in Guinness World Records.

Resilience and ikigai

If you have a clearly defined ikigai, you have one thing in common: you follow your passion, no matter what happens; they never give up, even when the odds seem to be against them or when they encounter one obstacle after another. However, resilience is more than just the ability to resist. As we will see in this chapter, it is also an attitude that we can develop to stay focused on the essential things in life and avoid being swept away by unpleasant feelings.

We will all encounter difficult situations at some point in our lives. The way we react to adversity will significantly affect our quality of life. Proper preparation is essential to deal with the ups and downs of life.

> Nana korobi ya oki 七転び八起き
> *Fall seven times, get up eight.*
>
> —Japanese proverb

The more resilient we are, the easier it will be to recover and return to what gives purpose to our lives.

Resilient individuals know how to stay focused on their goals, on what is essential, without succumbing to despair. Their flexibility is the foundation of their strength; they understand how to adjust to change and obstacles, even after making several blunders. Their flexibility is the foundation of their strength; they know how to adapt to change and obstacles, even after making many blunders. They focus on what they can control and don't care about what they can't. I'll give you the example of Derek Redmond. In Barcelona 1992, In an unforgettable semifinal of the 400m, During the semifinal of the 400 meters flat, the American Derek Redmond tears the biceps femoris of the right leg.

Despite everything, he decides to finish the race, and to help him in the effort comes his father, who comes down from the stands and enters the track passing the security personnel.

Father and son conclude the race together, and the public gives them the proper ovation.

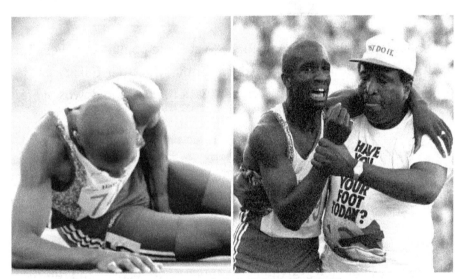

A STORY OF RESILIENCE

African-American pilot Bessie Coleman became the first black woman authorized to fly a commercial aircraft in the United States. In the early 1900s, this poor black lady lived in a society perpetuated by racism toward skin color and intolerance toward women. This ordinary person, who starts from a poor condition, turns into a celebrity of aerobatic flight in opposition to the discriminatory legislation of the time.

He worked for a starving pay as a manicure employee in Chicago, where he served wealthy clients. She is 23 years old when after listening to the many combat stories of pilots returning from the First World War, she developed a strong interest in aviation and became a professional pilot. Bessie, who grew up on a cotton farm in Texas, was able to test the devastating strength of resilience.

Her first efforts to learn to fly were a complete and total disaster, enough to discourage anyone with a modicum of common sense, **but not her.**

All the instructors, the flight schools, the social rules, even common sense were against her. After a thousand difficulties, she managed to apply to a specialized institute; She was escorted to the door on time because she was a woman and because she was black. His economic condition did not help; all the elements were against her, it seemed that all the facts were in agreement in preventing the realization of her dream. He had nothing but a strong determination and an unwavering faith.

When we refuse to give up, Dio himself puts himself on our side to move the mountains

If losing is a matter of persisting and believing against all reasoning and counter-force, this woman's life demonstrates that resilience mixed with confidence can move mountains. In recognition of her tenacity and faith, she was awarded a scholarship to continue her studies in France.

A legendary character was born, a woman capable of accomplishing feats unthinkable even for many men. He died in a plane crash at 34, leaving a touching testimony of courage and dedication.

The present and the impermanence of things

Knowing when the right time is coming is another critical aspect of resilience development. The present is the only thing we partially have control over. Opportunities are like open doors; they open and close if you don't enter on time. Without stressing about the past or the future that doesn't belong to us, we should grab things now. Put your mind: **Anxiety lives in the future, depression in the past.**

We must never forget that everything we own and everyone we care about will disappear at some point; we must be grateful for what we have had and **seize every opportunity today** while the doors are open.

"Human things are fleeting and perishable," says Seneca.

In the West, we have become accustomed to the stability of stone structures, which gives us the impression that nothing changes, making us forget the passage of time. Greco-Roman architecture loves symmetry, sharp lines, imposing facades, and structures resistant to the test of time.

"Nothing is created, nothing is destroyed, everything is transformed?"

Apart from the fact that man is a creature insofar as he is created, he does not escape this rule for the rest. Man does not destroy himself but changes, "transforms" what will become of him after the so-called earthly life? As for the body, we know that a rapid transformation occurs due to the cessation of vital activities. Medical science defines a person as clinically dead if one or both of the following clinical conditions occur:

1. The irreversible loss of cardiovascular and respiratory functions.
2. Or an Irreversible loss of all brain functions, including the brain stem.

These statements are exact when defining the process. Unfortunately, these definitions lack some essential basic principles. Without an authentic, deep, personal, and revealing experience, we will not be able to reach our Ikigai.

What, then, will become the center of existence? Feelings? Life experiences? of memories? Of the affections? And private property? And of us as eternal souls? We will have to take a step back and get to the origin; we will do it later.

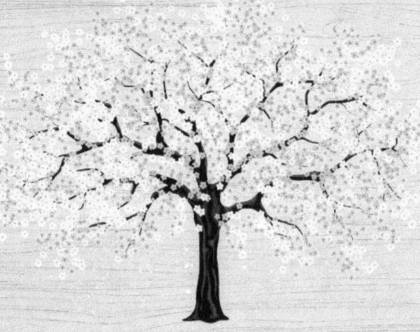

LET'S RENEW OUR MIND

BE TRANSFORMED BY THE RENEWAL OF YOUR MIND

The mind is the first battlefield

S hlomo Breznitz is an Israeli neurologist; He believes that the brain needs to exercise in a certain way to stay in shape. Breznitz says **the brain fosters more clear thinking by using shortcuts.** When a problem is presented, we can study it to discover a new solution or draw on previous experiences. The first process is tedious but can produce new ideas and leads to ikigai. The second option is simple and automatic and inspires confidence. However, depending on experience could make us overlook essential elements. The solution you used earlier may not work. In addition, **depending on occasion does not stimulate the brain to new connections.**

In neuroscience and biology, the **phrase neural network refers** to a dense network or circuit composed of neurons. Neural networks are defined as groupings of neurons that perform a particular physiological function.

The biological network uses many fundamental computational units (neurons) densely connected to change their structure in response to new external inputs: learning; when learning, new neural networks are created.

Three fundamental

components make up a neuron

1. The primary structure of the cell is **soma**.
2. **The axon** is the line of passage of every single neuron that branches into large amounts of branches.
3. The entry line is **dendrite**, which receives signals from other axons through synapses.

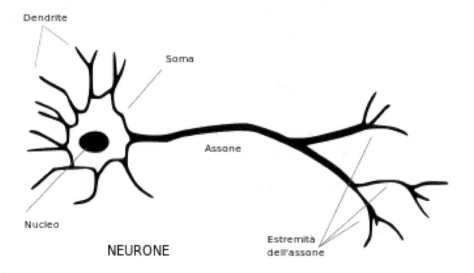

NEURONE

The cell body evaluates incoming signals. If the result exceeds a specific threshold value, the neuron is activated, and an "action potential" is produced, which is then transferred to the axon. If the result does not exceed the threshold value, the neuron remains resting.

Humans were created with a creative mind and an infinite imagination; this allows an intense use of the neural network and consequently new neural connections, keeping the brain young. Unbelievably vast are the resources of a mind regenerated and guided by the creator's spirit. However, there is a conflict between what is best and what we do; this is due mainly because many people, especially the elderly, prefer to do things the way they have always done them. Too much habit does not allow the brain to create new neural connections, favoring aging.

When the brain is exposed to new knowledge, it forms new connections and regenerates. However, exposing yourself to constant change can create stress because you leave your comfort zone.

Being us spiritual beings, as we will see later, the mind is involved despite ourselves in a spiritual fight that begins in our thoughts. When it happens to pass dark and dejection periods, a whirlwind of uncontrolled negative reviews seems to pass through our minds, which produce destructive feelings, such as depression and anxiety.

We are probably going through a spiritual attack that affects the mind, spirit, and body. We cannot leave our intellect in a passive state; passivity is the enemy of our ikigai, we must react.

We cannot prevent birds, understood as thoughts, from flying over our heads, but we can prevent them from nesting and making our condition.

The good news is that we are armed, and we can demolish reasoning and all that rises with pride against actual knowledge, making every thought prisoner until it is made obedient.

Here are some weapons at our disposal that we can use effectively:

1. **The word, if used against any adverse situation.** With the same principle that the world was created through the word, the term can be a weapon because it possesses creative power. Even better if we repeat with feeling, faith, and emotion words and promises made by the creator.
2. **Speaking clearly and directly** to situations, the one that comes, has a powerful impact if the request is made with confidence and without a doubt.
3. **Should we be reading positive** literature **that keeps, the mind engaged.** As we read, our faith increases because faith comes from the word, in this case, by reading; therefore, a positive reading is recommended as it could be to read La Tōrāh, the Hebrew book containing the Pentateuch exists in the American version.

These principles are essential to achieve your Ikigai; you will be surprised by the changes if you start practicing to use these weapons consistently.

I want to make sure you can understand what I mean. Faith is that essential component to grasp something invisible but not for this reason not real.

- Invisible does **not** necessarily **mean** non-existent.

You cannot find your Ikigai without faith. When we use the word of faith, we also use creative power.

Simply put, what you say with faith will happen. I have strived to have faith; I wanted to produce a feeling of trust and certainty for a matter that I wanted to change. I kept repeating positive words like "I have faith that something is happening." Unfortunately, as much as I tried not to listen to my heart, my feelings and my deep heart thought remained in the position of disbelief. Insisting on repeating positive words was useless. Until one day, I realized something significant. Listen well to what I will tell you because it is not something theoretical.

1. FAITH COMES FROM TO HEARING
2. HEARING COMES FROM THE WORD OF GOD
3. FAITH MUST BE CREDIBLE TO YOU

You cannot rest your faith on something abstract that you find unrealizable. These three points mean that you will never believe something that is not logical to you; you will not be able to make something logical and credible if you do not first repeatedly hear the word. When you have heard enough about what you want to take, then faith and the feeling of trust will naturally come without any effort, will be strong enough to move mountains, and will not need help. Essa will flow powerfully into your life, like a robust high-voltage cable; it will connect you to the God of the invisible, the power-producing power center necessary to grasp the invisible, making you take what you need.

The faith works **in this order; listen first, become credible later, and finally, flow. When it has released its flow, Faith will produce the materialization of the object of our request.** Once we receive an answer to our faith, we will create what I call the experience of faith, which will be a kind of cement that will strengthen your future faith.

If there is something, you wish to change, no matter how difficult it is, no matter that there is no hope, you can change this situation now by applying faith correctly.

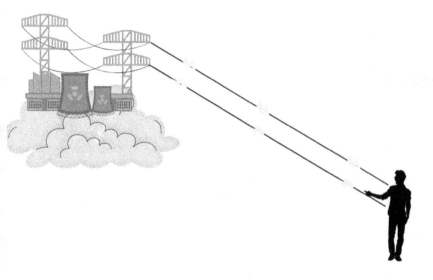

The search for meaning

Viktor Frankl, born in Vienna, 26/03/1905 and died in Vienna, 2 /09 /1997, was a neurologist, psychiatrist, philosopher, father, and founder of existential analysis and logotherapy. This method tends to highlight the individual's profoundly human and spiritual core. The search for meaning became a personal driving force in Frankl's life, allowing him to achieve specific goals.

However, this discipline is partial because it ignores the spirit's needs; **These five steps can be used to describe the process of logotherapy:**

1. A person feels impoverished, irritated, or worried.

2. The therapist shows him that he feels the expressed desire to live a meaningful life.

3. The sufferer finds the meaning of his existence (at that particular moment).

4. The patient chooses to accept or reject his destiny of free choice passively.

5. His renewed enthusiasm for life helps him overcome difficulties and sorrows.

On the other hand, Frankl was willing to risk his life to uphold his moral principles. Auschwitz taught him that man has the faculty to choose his path in any circumstance, using the faculty of free will. That experience inspired him for the rest of his life.

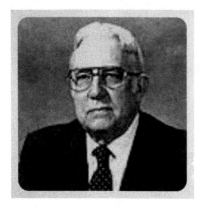

The history of Charles Edward Greenaway, indifferently from religious and political beliefs, shows an example of meaning very clearly. He founded the ADI congregations in Burkina Faso, Togo, Benin, and Senegal; He dedicated his life to missions in these states. This man worked hard for years, in health conditions Precarious and with a large part of the heart no longer working. The doctors had said that he could no longer do the missionary, who would die if he had left again, but he did not listen because he had a call "ikigai" very strong. One day during a visit, a physician stated, "*this man lives only for the strong motivation that possesses, stop it equivale to make him die.*"

BELOW IS A BRIEF EXCERPT OF HIS MANY STORIES:

A burning desire can extend life expectancy. "... In 1946, I was dying of black fever, in a dirty house in Burkina Faso. Previously, I had counted 126 burials of missionaries under forty in West Africa. I buried my friends and looked at the bodies of those who had died on my lap just moments before. Lord, why! I shouted. Every time I left a tomb, I knew they had killed to proclaim the King's death, resurrection, and return (Jesus).

I was in the hut, bleeding, sluggish, with a horrible fever, without hope, doctors, medication, and other missionaries, just me and my wife. "Charles, we have done all that God has commanded us to do, we have thrown bread on the rivers, He will come, the bread will come back to us," she continued as tears ran down her cheeks.

Then he heard in the distance singing: "There is power in the blood of Jesus, power! Power! The precious blood of Jesus has power!"

"The angels in the choir of heaven welcome me," I shouted to my wife.

The tam-tams were playing, and everyone was singing, "There is power in the blood of Jesus."

Who was he? They were the bread we threw away.

The tribes we had spoken to earlier. The chief said, madam, her husband, he came, he taught us about Jesus, and we were saved, he told us about baptism in the Holy Spirit, and we were baptized, he told us about healing, and God healed many of us, we never prayed for anyone, but we would pray for him, they said my wife. These men began to pray on the dirty floor surrounding my bed, and their pleas reached heaven. God looked down from the gates of glory and observed to the angels: "It's Greenaway."

God knows us. God is present at the smallest burial of the bird. God knows us and calls us! God offers infinite grace, hope, and the most excellent doctor when He opens His hand. He sent me his Power and I was completely healed!

When those people saw me, a scream of triumph rose to heaven, the tam-tams began to play again, and everyone sang.

We had visitors for two days and two nights. Our modest cottage attracted the city."

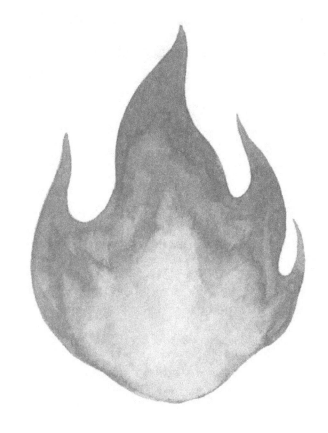

A burning desire

Another new element has been added to faith, the ardent desire. Burning desire is much more than a positive feeling or attitude. All of us have longed for something we couldn't have in our lives; to achieve something that we have desired always involves paying the price, the more critical this thing is to succeed, the higher the price, it is so in trade, and so in the world, and so also in the spiritual Kingdom.

Many times, as I think I will have happened to you, I had to be content to resize my desire by finding the right compromise between price and desire for fulfillment.

Who among us has never happened to want a nice car but to have bought a less expensive one, having to settle?

The answer is obvious; it is because of the price. The best car has a higher price. There is a close correlation between price (or cost) and result. There is no result without a fee, and there is no price paid that does not produce the result.

I understand that what I am about to say may be considered foolish to many. Why didn't I buy the best car? For lack of money?

- **No, for the lack of an ardent desire.**

Do you think it is possible to stop a person who lives only and exclusively to achieve his goal?

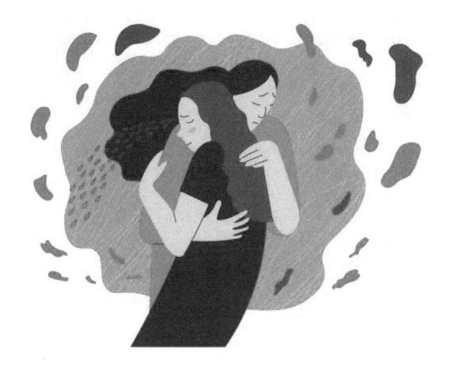

Existential satisfaction

Existential dissatisfaction occurs when our lives seem to have no meaning, our purpose is distorted, and we do not hear our call (ikigai).

Logotherapy sees this dissatisfaction as deep anguish, a natural event that motivates people who suffer from it to seek a solution and, in doing so, to discover a greater appreciation for life.

Existential crises have always existed in every age. Individuals do what they are instructed to do or what others do, rather than what they wish to do.

Sunday neurosis, for example, occurs when a person discovers how empty he feels inside without the responsibilities and commitments of the work week. It must find a solution. Above all, he must find out his purpose, his reason for getting out of bed - his ikigai.

It seems that man has within him a void with a particular form.

Many ignore that the nature of this need is spiritual. Men Try to fill it through material things, such as cars, houses, jewelry, money, and luxury. But all these goods cannot satisfy the existential void precisely because they are material in nature and not spiritual. We will explain these concepts in more detail in a transparent way.

"I FEEL EMPTY INSIDE"

Frankl's group showed that many of the patients interviewed in research at the Vienna Polyclinic Hospital suffered from an existential crisis.

This great scholar has done an excellent job of showing that man is in search of completeness and inner peace. The human being comes to a child who seeks his father; he looks for himself. Failure to achieve his life purpose makes man disappointed, sad, and dissatisfied.

Watching many individuals lead happy and entire lives over time, I realized that the profound inner emptiness is a universal experience.

World War II

The racist and oppressive policies of the Nazi regime lasted from 1933 to 1945 and forced millions of people to fight for their lives. Of the approximately 17 million victims of the Holocaust (including 6 million Jews), the survivors were a minority. **Meno of a third of the nine million European Jews.**

Unfortunately, the world war is one of the saddest and darkest pages of the whole of humanity. We must be cautious as humans because cycles tend to repeat themselves, and the limitations on freedom gradually move on to extermination.

During this period of detention, psychiatrists found that the inmates who had the best chance of surviving in German concentration camps **had goals to achieve outside the base and possessed a strong desire to live**; this was true for Frankl; he successfully founded his school after being freed.

Frankl's persistence was motivated by a specific purpose; he had created a document that included all the thoughts and research of his career and was about to publish it before arriving at Auschwitz. When it was confiscated from him, to cope with the continuous terror and uncertainty of life in the concentration camp, he used any piece of paper he could get his hands on and brought back on them, part of the lost work, until he reassembled it.

Forgiveness case study

A prominent U.S. ambassador went to Frankl for a course of therapy he had begun five years earlier. When Frankl asked why he had started treatment in the first place, the ambassador reported that he despised his work and his country's foreign policies. The ambassador was on terrible terms with his father, but his psychotherapist urged him to make peace.

For a time, the ambassador refused, continuing to live in frustration and despising his job, but when the ambassador decided to forgive unconditionally, he experienced indescribable peace and joy. Lack of forgiveness causes frustration and pain; a person closed in his distress is caged inside by a dark wall, which remains impassable. Esso swallows up all joy, peace, and satisfaction. Life is often unfair, and it is accessible to harbor hatred, resentment, and disappointment.

Our reaction determines whether or not we will overcome that adversity.

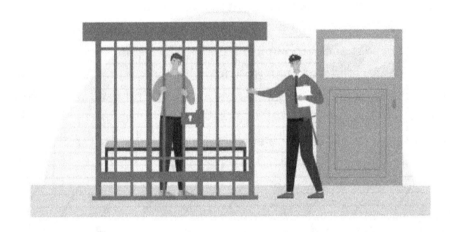

A person who hates, is free, or is an enslaved person?

Who hates has a feeling that grows and **requires more and more space**. The lack of forgiveness like a monster grows and deprives the unfortunate of all the joy of living, of seeing one's children grow up, enjoying simple things, and having peace.

Usually, the excuses of non-forgiveness are:

- **It hurt me too much!**
- **It is not possible to forgive in such cases!**
- **I had given him everything, and he betrayed me!**

Forgiveness as a cure

One of the arguments we frequently use when "forgiving" is."**I forgave him, but**" he must come first to apologize.

- I forgave him, **but** he will no longer be able to enter my house!
- I forgave him, **but** I can't get him back!
- I have forgiven him, **but** certain things are unforgettable!

We are looking for the real ikigai, so it needs me to be honest and tell you how exactly things are:

- It is necessary to pass from forgiveness; it is impossible to find peace without it. Stability is required to live long and well

Forgiveness on the creator's part is subordinate to the forgiveness that man must offer to his neighbor. This principle explains very well in the following story:

One day a King decided to come to terms with his servants. He was presented with the case of a servant who owed him ten thousand talents when the accounts began. (*Era an unpayable debt.!!!!*) However, since he did not have the talents to repay the loan, the master ordered it be sold together with his wife, children, and assets to repay the debt. The servant, who had been thrown to the ground, then pleaded with him, saying, "*My Lord, be patient with me, and I will give you back everything.*" The master was sorry for the condition of the servant, then he allowed him to go and canceled his debt. As soon as he came out, however, the servant looked for another of his preserves, who owed him only a hundred denarii, and suffocated him, saying:

"Pay what you owe!" When he was thrown to the ground, his friend begged him, saying:

"*Have a little patience, and I will repay the debt.*" But, since he refused to listen, he had him imprisoned until the amount was paid all.

When the other servants saw what was happening, they were outraged and rushed to inform their lord.

The King then brought that servant and said, "Wicked servant, I have forgiven you all your debts because you pleaded with me, and I had compassion."

Didn't you also have compassion for your friend?

And, outraged, the master entrusted him to the guards and went to prison until he had repaid all the debts.

If you do not forgive heartily, you will be given pride guards, and you will find yourself in a prison of resentment, anger, and resentment.

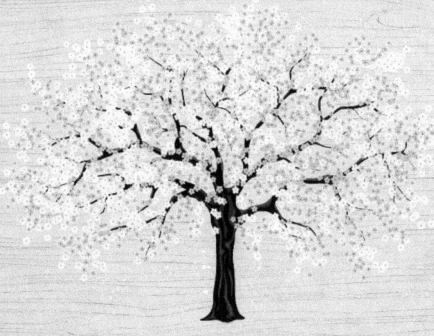

THE POWER OF FORGIVENESS

BECAUSE IF YOU FORGIVE MEN THEIR SINS, YOUR HEAVENLY FATHER WILL FORGIVE YOU TOO.

True forgiveness and ikigai

Several psychological investigations and research projects have shown that forgiveness is beneficial for one's physical, emotional, and social state. Forgiving has a positive impact on health and happiness.

The benefits of body forgiveness include **reducing heart rate** and **blood pressure and reducing cortisol levels,** and consequently lower stress levels. It also helps with insomnia, relieves discomfort, and prevents migraines by strengthening the immune system.

On a psychological level, forgiving is beneficial because **it increases our self-esteem reduces depressive symptoms and anxiety.** It makes us more empathetic, patient, less inflexible, and more tolerant.

Forgiveness also has social benefits, such as improving bonds with family, fathers and sons, siblings, and even spouses and facilitating father-child connections.

But what is true forgiveness? True ikigai leads to forgiveness. **The quality of our forgiveness is critical** to achieving true peace. Let's not settle for surrogates like that; I forgave "but."

Forgiveness is symbolized by two Greek terms that have specific connotations:

1. The first is **Aphiemi,** which means to release, dissolve, set free, renounce and provide someone or something.
2. The Greek term **Hilaskomai,** on the other hand, has a specific connotation. Atonement, reconciliation, and they are all

beneficial. To conciliate oneself, to appease the wrathful God.

The term consists of three main actors:

- The One who **forgives**
- The One Who Receives Forgiveness
- The creator **guarantor** and judge, on the laws that govern forgiveness

So it follows that: when we forgive, we **release from the chains**, we dissolve a bond, and we renounce any present, past, and future claim, permanently, abandoning any revenge or feeling connected to it. **But who is in chains?** The answer is simple: both those in debt and those who wait for payment are in prison. As a result of forgiveness, the situation is dead, forgotten, and everything returns to its original state, so forgiving the creator does not accept lower standards; those who receive forgiveness are also **freed from the weight of a conscience** occupied by debt and the consequences that derive from it; however, he is obliged by universal law to maintain the same attitude towards others.

The creator is the first to bestow forgiveness and does not ask for a replacement. Since the debt could not be paid, he Practically forgives each person using the payment made by his son, regardless of how high our debt is. Murder, adultery, theft, greed, and forgiveness overflows with the law of offense.

The creator on condition that one addresses him personally, without other mediators than his son, with a sincere and repentant heart, free from the tormentors of guilt, from an oppressed and condemned mind. He will regenerate our minds, freeing the soul from all burdens.

I invite you to experience the power of forgiveness, forgive by turning to the creator and then go to those who have wronged you and forgive him; if you do it sincerely, you will feel a very powerful ikigai.

How we can excel

We excel at what we repeatedly do. Excellence, therefore, is not an act but a habit.

—Aristotle

Let's say you're skiing on one of your favorite slopes. The snow flakes fall abundantly. The conditions are ideal.

You know exactly how to ski; you don't think about the future or the past. You use snow, skis, body, and mind for one thing; this is the correct attitude when we want to find the true purpose of life.

We've all had the feeling that time flies when we're involved in an activity we love. When we spend a day reading a book, we are unaware of the passage of time until we see the sunset and realize that we have not had dinner.

But **if we have to do something we don't want, every minute will feel like an eternity,** and we can't stop looking at our watches. "Put your hand on a hot burner for a minute, and it will look like an hour," Einstein is said to have said. Being with your beloved for an hour seems like a minute; this is the concept of relativity. "

What makes us love something so much that we forget everything while doing it? When are we happiest? **We must continue to seek tirelessly, with all the soul, mind, and the whole body; this is the only way to seek the truth.**

Feelings

Since feelings come from the heart and are guided by what we pay most attention to, we deduce from them that "where your treasure is, it will also be your heart."

Feelings cannot be controlled directly; they do not obey. Just as the heart cannot increase the beats to our liking, the emotions also work similarly.

Ignorance on these points is a contributing cause of failure. Many people know that they should eat healthier and lose weight, would like to quit smoking, do something better, or simply want to feel better people.

Although we cannot act directly on the heart to tell it to speed up or slow down, **we can act indirectly to control it.**

If we wanted to speed it up, it would be enough to walk or run; similarly, to make it slow down, it would be enough to rest. So our feelings are influenced by what we watch and do for a long time a day, and eventually, that thing will end up being in our hearts and guiding our feelings.

If you repeatedly direct **your mind, readings, and actions on sweet, pure, and virtuous things, your heart will be directed towards these things with their feelings, and you will find their virtues.**

Creativity

Mihaly Csikszentmihalyi, a Hungarian psychologist born in the early 900s. He defined the feeling of being completely absorbed in what we are doing **as "flow".**

To achieve this optimal experience, **we must take care** of **the quantity and quality of time we devote to activities that bring us into this state,** rather than allowing ourselves to be absorbed in activities that provide immediate pleasure, such as consuming a lot of food, drug or alcohol abuse, wasting time on social media.

As Csikszentmihalyi states, **flow is "the condition in which people are so involved in an activity that nothing else seems to matter;**

Not only creative workers need high levels of attention to create. Most sportsmen, chess players and engineers also devote a significant amount of their time to things that push them to this condition.

According to research, **a chess player feels the same way as a mathematician** working on a formula or a surgeon performing an operation.

But what happens to our minds when we reach that point?

When, we are completely absorbed in a certain activity without distractions. Our minds are "in order." The opposite happens when we try to do something while our mind is on other things, leaving the mind passive is equivalent to leaving it in disorder.

The creator with immense creative potential designed the human mind. Still, often this valuable tool is left at the mercy of social networks, digital games, and other things that serve to entertain the person constantly. Entertainment is the enemy of order and flow.

The following conditions must be met to reach the flow:

1. Be aware of what to do
2. Understanding how to make it happen
3. Understand how well you are doing. Know where to go (navigation is involved)
4. Perceiving substantial difficulties
5. Recognize important skills
6. The absence of distractions

Here's how social media affects our brains:

Most users cannot manage their time falling into a real addiction, con mechanisms similar to those of drugs. Some studies have caused a deterioration of white matter in regions that regulate emotions, attention, and decisions. That instant gratification provided by social media leads the brain to develop an addiction to the stimulation that dopamine provides.

People who spend a lot of time on social media are less adept at being able to change activities.One survey found that 89% of respondents

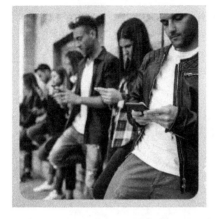 had the perception of receiving notifications even with the phone turned off.

A cause of social media. The regions of the brain that evaluate tactile sensations,   like the bark somato-sensory Perceive stimuli Electronic What "ghost limbs" who they interfere with our tactile impressions. DOPAMINE, the reward regions of the brain are more engaged on social media, so dopamine is produced, a chemical linked to the emotions of well-being that is addictive and asks for more and more stimulus.

The University of Chicago has found that   online interpersonal connections exceed real ones.

Element 1
Practice a moderate activity

The approach of Schaffer, a psychologist born in Berlin in 1926 from a Jewish family, was one of the essential developmental psychologists in the United Kingdom. He urges us to undertake **activities that we believe we can do but that are outside our comfort zone.**

The comfort zone is represented for our brain by a series of standard rules that tend to repeat themselves almost automatically over time and prevent us from finding new solutions.

Every sport or profession has rules that require many skills. We are prone to getting bored if the rules for accomplishing a job or achieving a goal are too simple compared to our skill set. **Too simple activities cause apathy.**

If, on the other hand, we set ourselves too hard a goal, we will lack the necessary skills, and **we will probably stop feeling irritated.**

The ideal situation is to find a middle path that falls within our capabilities but with moderate difficulty, to see it as an affordable challenge. When Ernest Hemingway remarked, "Sometimes I write better than I can," he meant that.

We want to overcome difficulties because we love the feeling of pushing ourselves further. Bertrand Russell said:

"Being able to concentrate for a significant period of time is necessary for a difficult realization."

Learn a new software application for your next project if you are a graphic designer. Use a new programming language if you are a programmer.

Add something special, something that pushes you out of your comfort zone

Even something as basic as reading requires the application of specific principles and the possession of particular skills and information. If we started reading a book on quantum mechanics for physicists without being one, we would probably give up in a few minutes. Even though we already know everything a reader has to offer, we'll quickly get bored.

However, if the book is relevant to our knowledge and skills and adds to what we already know, we will immerse ourselves in our reading, and time will fly by.

Set a specific and measurable goal

TBoard games and sports are excellent methods of creating flow since the goal is usually quite clear: **to beat your opponent while using a set of well-established guidelines.**

According to a survey by the Boston Consulting Group, **workers' complaints about their managers is that they don't "convey a goal to the team,"** as a result, employees don't know what exactly to do.

Executives engage in obsessive planning devising methods but lack a clear goal. It's like setting sail with a map but without any destination.

It is more important to have a compass pointing to a goal rather than having a map. A compass will always lead you in the right direction.

"Who among you, wanting to build a tower, does not sit down first to calculate its expense if you have the means to complete it? To avoid that, if he lays the foundation and cannot finish the work, everyone who sees it begins to mock him, saying: He began to build, but he could not complete the job. "

Before you start working, study, or create anything;

it is essential to think about what we want to achieve and set a goal.

We should ask ourselves questions like, "What is my goal for today's study session? "

For a little or for a long time

Having a clear goal is essential to achieving the flow, but we also need to know how to leave it behind when we get to work. Once the journey begins, we should keep this goal in mind without being obsessed with it.

When Olympic competitors compete for gold medals, they can't help but notice how attractive the prize is. But they must be present at the moment of athletic performance.

If they lose concentration for a fraction of a second, they will make a mistake and forfeit the prize.

A fraction of a second is a minimal, almost insignificant value; we can be tempted to overlook it. But it is a very significant value when it makes us lose the prize.

Do not neglect the day of small things. Precision in small things will bring you precision in big things.

The question we have to ask ourselves is, am I running so that I bring back my prize? Do I know what the rules are?

Life, therefore, has its own rules and its higher purpose, and it has a motive and a logic. Thus, ignorance of these laws will not protect us because the law does not admit ignorance.

The Roman procurator Phaistos met Paul to question him about his beliefs. While Paul precisely expounded his doctrine and purpose of life, Festus found himself interested in admiring such a lively faith and an unusual motivation. Festus was fascinated by Paul and what he represented.

Hence the famous phrase *"for a short time or Paul do not convince me to be yours."*

It makes no difference for a little or a long measure; the little things make us lose or achieve the big stuff. The good is the enemy of the best.

Japanese Takumi

Steve Jobs, the co-founder of Apple, was a great admirer of Japan. He was fascinated by the simplicity and quality of Japanese porcelain; when he visited Sony in 1980, he adopted many of their techniques.

Un Takumi (匠"craftsman" or 巧"expert") named Yukio Shakunaga employed a unique artisanal method, Etchu Seto-yaki, which earned the love of Steve Jobs.

During a trip to Kyoto, Jobs learned about an exhibition of Shakunaga's art. He immediately saw that Shakunaga porcelain was unique.

Jobs went to Kyoto many times during his lifetime searching for inspiration and eventually met Shakunaga in person. According to legend, Jobs had numerous questions for him, almost all of them concerned the production method and the type of porcelain he used.

So far, Shakunaga claims to be the only artist of his kind who knows the entire process of making porcelain objects, from their origins in the mountains to their ultimate form, a genuinely unique Takumi.

You have to try to be unique when you do something. Not to be competitive, but creative. You will get out of stress and do better.

Jobs was so impressed that he thought of going to Toyama to visit the mountain from where Shakunaga got his porcelain but decided not to do so after learning that it was more than four hours by train from Kyoto.

Shakunaga said in an interview after Jobs' death that he was honored that his effort was recognized by the brilliant guy who invented the iPhone.

Simplicity as the key

As Csikszentmihalyi would argue, the key to maintaining constant flow has a significant task to complete.

Another example of Takumi, this time in the kitchen, can be seen in the documentary Jiro Dreams of Sushi. Its main character has been cooking sushi every day for over eighty years and runs a small sushi restaurant near Tokyo's Ginza subway station. He perfected himself beyond all limits by carrying out the same gestures every day, apparently repetitive and straightforward.

The brain learns by making mistakes and repeating to the bitter end

He and his son go to the renowned Tsukiji Fish Market every day to choose the most acceptable catch to bring back to the restaurant.

In the film, we witness several scenes where one of Jiro's students learns to do something seemingly simple, create the Tamago (a thin and slightly sweet omelet). Despite several attempts, he will not gain Jiro's approval. He practices for years without getting tired until finally, his master approves of him.

What is the motivation of the apprentice who made him refuse to surrender when it was logical to do so?

Isn't he tired of frying eggs every day? No, since he has a strong desire to succeed, that work coincided with his flow.

Even after earning a three-Michelin star rating, they never thought about opening more locations or growing the company.

Jiro, like Yukio Shakunaga, starts his work from the "source," always taking the information from the source and unfiltered. Shakunaga travels to the highlands to find the best porcelain, while Jiro goes to the fish market to get the best tuna.

Better teacher or teacher?

Master comes from Magis, which means "more," so the master is **"who is more"** in every situation. A teacher is someone who transmits his knowledge, which becomes the foundation of other professions. Simply put, a teacher has pupils and is someone who prepares students with notions suitable for a career, knowledge, or craft.

The teacher has disciples who want to follow in his footsteps, not only in the teaching but also in the life steps. The master merely stimulates the disciple. Only if he responds to this impulse the disciple comes to authentic learning; **otherwise, he will be** a pupil. A pupil would not have learned Jiro's lesson; a disciple would.

The nature of man

The original man was a pure and perfect creature; he had implanted the perfect ikigai by birth; the human form was akin to the image of the creator of all things and a supporter of every universal lectern. He was incapable of doing evil because his spirit was constantly in contact with the creator and reflected his perfection; since the nature of the creator is loving, the man was also caring. Therefore, he was not an Egocentric being, but Theocentric, thus representing the perfection that the creator reflected on nature.

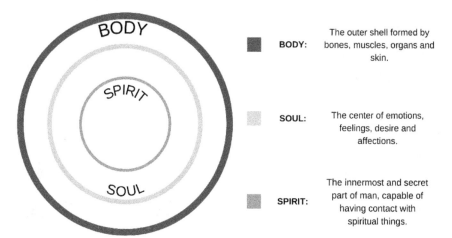

BODY: The outer shell formed by bones, muscles, organs and skin.

SOUL: The center of emotions, feelings, desire and affections.

SPIRIT: The innermost and secret part of man, capable of having contact with spiritual things.

The human being is essentially composed of three distinct components, but at the same time are part of the same person; as a bundle of roses composed of three roses, they are a single bunch and at the same time three different roses. The diagram below will give us a better understanding:

There is a potent force for which science has found no formal explanation. No one knows what it is, but it is a force that understands and manages all others.

This universal force is love.

— Albert Einstein

This great physicist of the twentieth century, known for the formula of mass-energy equivalence, $E = mc^2$, recognized as *"the most famous equation in the world,"* and for the law of relativity, gave a clear definition of the meaning of life and the achievement of one's Ikigai.

The interruption of the flow

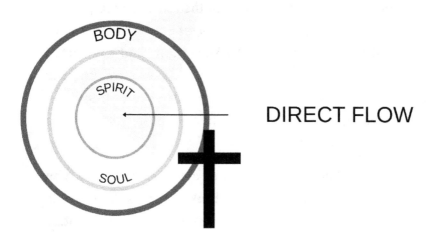

DIRECT FLOW

What interrupted the direct flow, creator of human perfection, longevity, and a motivated and prosperous fulfilled life? (ikigai)

THE VIOLATION OF UNIVERSAL LAW

When we violate the law, it is correct to expect a consequence; the more critical the norm, the greater the weight of the sentence, the more influential the one who establishes the standard, the greater the punishment. **Violations are also convicted.** The man received his salary, the *"condemnation"* to death, Regardless of how good people, respectable and religious, are thought to be.

Come is established for men who die only once, after which comes judgment.

The violation of the law entered the world because of one man, *(Hebrew: אָדָם?) 'dm means man, Adam.* We also find this fact mentioned in the Sumerian plates and the Bible.

The violation, seized the opportunity of the law has brought with it as a consequence death; in fact, the wages of sin is death. Since the law existed, there was no transgression, and one acted according to conscience, but the law gave strength and effectiveness to the violation and death that derives from it. It follows that death has passed on all men because of the nature inherited from the first man.

For all have sinned and are deprived of divine glory. Every man has violated the law when the first has broken it; it is as if the whole world to follow was in the loins of the first man who violated it.

When one nation declares war on another, the declaration includes men, women, present children, and future children, those who are aware of it and those who are not informed.

Man, having become non-spiritual, cannot change things, no human effort, made to mend the tear and sufficient.

One labors in matters and expects the divine verdict.

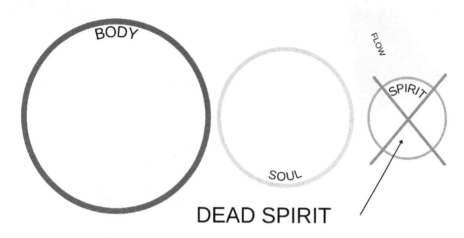

DEAD SPIRIT

— **Japanese Saying**

Every person born in that nation will be considered an enemy of the other, even if he has not declared war personally. **Death, however, did not manifest itself immediately in body and soul but did its work in the spirit first,** mortifying it and depriving it of the faculty of coming into contact with spiritual things. Man is no longer Theocentric but Egocentric and separated from his creator. For this reason, before one can find one's ikigai, the spirit must be revitalized and be able to grasp the true meaning of life again.

A unique love comes from heaven...

— Japanese Saying

The current condition

The wasted water *can no longer return to the tray*

— **Japanese Saying**

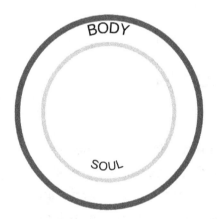

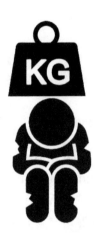

Love is that power that moves the universe, motivates man's life, gives a purpose. **But unfortunately, man has broken up and cannot give true love because he is devoid of it by nature, so he does not find the real Ikigai.** Now he lives with an existential burden that he cannot satisfy. You can repay damage, fix a chair, renew a piece of furniture. But as the water does not return to the tray, it **is** impossible to remedy the law's violation **since the law, even if the right has too high a price to pay.**

A man deprived of contact with the divine has become selfish, self-centered, empty; whatever activity he does, he cannot replace the emptiness left in his spirit because he is of another nature. Every human work is material. If therefore, the human being is not destroyed but transformed, he is an eternal being; consequently, the need for his ikigai to be maintained for eternity derives.

But he is far from his true purpose; he seeks it in material things, cars, money, success, but he realizes that nothing gives him what he seeks because nothing reaches his spirit to enliven it and make him find the true purpose life.

He feels a void but cannot fill it. He finds himself in an unconscious expectation that the second death will manifest itself on the body and its eternal soul.

The new life

"No one puts new wine in old wineskins; otherwise, the new wine bursts the skins, the wine spreads, and the skins are lost. But the new wine must be put in new wineskins.

And no one, who has drunk old wine, wants new wine, because he says: 'The old is good'".

This ancient parable speaks of:

- Old wineskins represent the old Adamic nature of man *"who is at war with his creator."*

- The **new skins** similarly represent the new nature received through the second Adam.

- The new wine represents the new spiritual life.

- **Old wine** represents the old way of living self-centered.

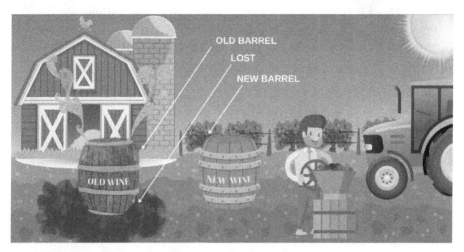

Nature is always the key to interpretation. The story's meaning is that the natural older man cannot receive new things and the life of the spirit remains unknown to him because his heart is not animated.

Moreover, with his way of thinking, the older man considers the new life madness, prefers the old wine or vitality that he has always drunk, does not want to leave his comfort zone, and does not want to create new connections. Those who have received the unique nature can receive the spirit's wine and preserve it because they can acquire and preserve it.

But those who have kept the old nature cannot receive the new things because they cannot do so and prefer the old wine.

Being a natural problem is not something related to doing what is right or what is wrong. You don't even need a lot of things to do since it's not a matter of crossing a certain threshold to become spiritual. By faith, we have been grafted on and have become partakers of the root and sap of the tree.

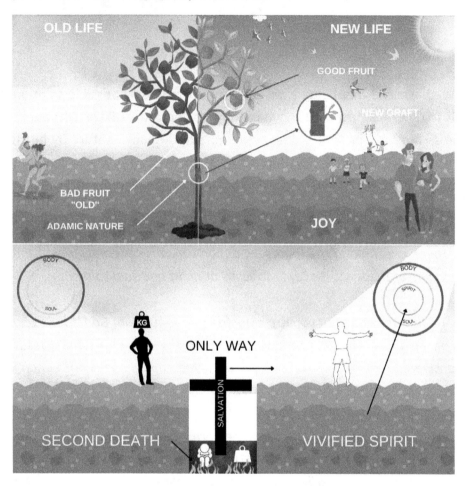

Receiving a new life

We have said that being a natural problem, the only possible solution is to receive a new nature; we cannot reach our true ikigai without it. Yes, but how to do it? Just as we inherited Adam's nature by birth, we should inherit a new nature by birth. We will have to be born precisely again. Now let someone higher than me explain to you what I mean:

"There was among the Pharisees a man called Nicodemus, one of the leaders of the Jews. He came to Jesus at night and said to him:

"Rabbi, we know that you are a doctor who came from God, for no one can do these miracles that you do if God is not with him." Jesus answered him, "Verily, verily, I say unto you, unless one is born again, he cannot see the kingdom of God."

Nicodemus said, "How can a man be born when he is already old? Can he enter his mother's womb a second time and be born?" Jesus answered, "Verily, verily, I say unto you, unless one is born of water and the Spirit, he cannot enter the kingdom of God. That which is born of the flesh "Adam" is flesh, and that which is born of the Spirit is spirit. Don't be surprised if I told you, "You need to be born again."

Nicodemus replied and said to him:

"How can these things happen?" Jesus answered him: "You are the teacher of Israel, and you do not know these things? Truly, I say that we speak of what we know and testify of what we have seen; but you do not receive our testimony. If I have spoken to you of earthly things and do not believe, how will you believe if I speak to you of heavenly things? No one has ascended to heaven, except the one who came down from heaven: the Son of man."

... "And just as Moses lifted the serpent in the wilderness, so the Son of man (Jesus) must be lifted, *that whoever believes in him may have eternal life.*

Because God so loved the world, that he gave his only begotten Son *so that whoever believes* in him may not perish but have eternal life. Infatuated, God did not send his Son into the world to judge the world but so that the world might be saved through him. **He who believes in him is not judged; he who does not believe is already judged** because he has not believed in the name of the only begotten Son of God.

The judgment is this: the light came into the world, and men preferred darkness to light because their works were evil. For whoever does bad things hates the light and does not come to light, so that his works may not be discovered; but whoever puts the truth into practice comes to light, so that his works may be manifested because they are made in God".

In this story, despite being a highly educated and mentally skilled man, Nicodemus could not understand that the new birth had to be spiritual. He wondered how it was possible to enter his mother's womb again; this is a practical example of how the natural person (Adam) cannot receive spiritual things.

Later his eyes were opened to "see" spiritual reality.

Having believed the words of Jesus, who would soon die in his place on the cross, to make the promise valid, Nicodemus **received a life-giving spirit or new life.**

The very moment he believed, he became able to understand spiritual realities and be freed from the judgment that was reserved for the old nature inherited from Adam.

Once again, the beautiful children come to the rescue of us adults. Because of their harmless purity, they have free access to the creator; children are the closest thing to heaven that we have on earth; **let us love them, protect them, and set an example. Nicodemus looked for complications and could not understand, but the children just believed. If you tell a child,** *"jump from the table, I take you, "* *the child will do it instantly, without* any fear, he will jump convinced that his dad will take him. He is his father, The thought that his father may not take him does not touch him in the slightest. If we ask the same thing to an adult, he will begin to reason, wondering if what we ask falls within his logical schemes. The celestial Kingdom does not follow our logic. In the natural world, we first see, and then we believe. In the spiritual Realm, we first believe then "see." The meaning of faith is to **"see" what is invisible but exists.**

If you chose this book, it is because you are sincerely in search of the truth **and your true ikigai.** For this reason, feeling responsible, I cannot afford to present you with an accommodating, distorted, or partial reality. To build, we must first demolish the old, or would we build a house on the rubble? It would not be wise!! Do you light a fire on the ashes? No. Unfortunately, now you may not like what I will tell you, but if you are sincerely seeking your true purpose, you must be stubborn as a disciple to pass from below; these principles could change your eternal vision and not just today's. I ask you to read the following story carefully.

One day a man was in his countryside. When he cultivated, following a copious rain, he saw a large nugget of shiny gold sticking out of the ground on a path. The rain had brought her to the surface: the farmer. Felice and joyful, picked it up, cleaned it up and quickly put it in his pocket, left the unfinished work to go running to his village to the goldsmith.

As he posed the cockets, joyful and festive, he thought about how his life would soon change and how he could spend such a fortune. Nearby he met an ambulant merchant, who cons his camels, brought the precious goods from the East. This merchant sold valuable products, the elderly gentleman had always wanted to be his customer, but he had never been able to afford it.

So impatiently, he made the merchant stop, and almost knocking him down, he made him get off his camel. The peasant observed the exquisite merchandise and chose the best commodity in possession of the merchant; fine leathers, delicate linen fabrics, rare aromas, perfumes, and delicious spices worthy of a prince. The merchant for a moment closed the trunk and, in a hesitant voice, said. *"My friend, I don't know you; I can't give you my most precious mercy if you don't give me the money first."* The farmer then smiled with taste and pulled out of his pocket that great nugget bright and shiny, if well it was still dirty with earth. The merchant will risk himself in the face at the sun to see it. "Well," exclaimed the merchant. *"My friend, dear friend, a customer like you is welcome; I can do a particular treatment for my best customers. You will render the goods and pay me later when you have changed the gold. Today I will stay in the city, just sign a pledge contract. "*

The older man gladly accepted and ran happily with the merchandise on his shoulder to change his gold. But when he entered the goldsmith jumping and dancing, he said, "enjoy soul, *for you will have goods to satiate your soul forever." He* opened his pocket and gently pulled out the nugget. The goldsmith, with a careful eye, looked at the nugget. *"Humm... Let me see you closer,"* he exclaimed. Then, after carefully examining the nugget, the experienced goldsmith cried with mocking air.

"My friend, you couldn't recognize that it was pyrite and not a big nugget of gold." Chuckling then added, *"the pyrite and the fools' gold, of those who do not know how to recognize the truth."*

Disconsolate, the farmer exclaimed, "ahi me, what a cancellation, *I will not be able to have goods at will as I had thought."* Then he tied the pyrite to his belt and ran back to his field where he had met the shopkeeper of precious goods. Seeing him as he passed by with his camels, he prayed to him, crying and telling him, "here is your trunk *still closed, take back the goods."*

The merchant replied, "*My friend, it's too late, you had to think about it before, a contract is a contract; also, you have soiled the trunk with mud, the goods have been muddied, and I can no longer sell it. Mi, you will have to pay up to the last penny.*"

So the man sadly lost his house and the countryside to repay his debt.

I want to tell you now about the law of attraction—this rampant doctrine that aims to enrich, partially proposing some truths.

According to these principles, your thoughts will become a reality; that is, you can intensely attract what you think about if you can bring it into your subconscious with repetition.

Man would also be able to save himself. Yes, but keep from what? It is not specified from what to protect oneself; to save oneself, one needs to know from what.

We are using terms such as "he who sees everything,"; "the universal force,"; "a loving and benign force." Everything is focused on receiving gifts from this unspecified "force," now and for the present life, everything we desire. Having studied in detail the aspects concerning this doctrine, I have to ask you some questions.

Is it wise to receive a gift without knowing who the giver is?

Since "the universal force" is spiritual life, it is therefore found in a spiritual world, more vast and full of dangers than the material world.

Would you ever send a child on the most infamous streets of a city to run errands?

What discernment might the child have, and how would he assess what is right from what is a danger?

We have said that man is an eternal being and possesses a spirit, although it is not vivified; just as there are ages for man and degrees of maturity for our body, there are also ages and degrees of maturity for our spirit. In the beginning, we need pure spiritual milk.

Looking out without knowledge and protection in the spiritual world, will we find ourselves in the condition of believing gold, which in reality is not?

Many people will be able to replicate that they have achieved their goals and have a great mindset. Of course, the farmer also found gold. Have you ever seen someone buy more time with their money? "except for medical care that helps you live better and longer"

Has anyone ever brought with them the accumulated material goods?

As you pass away from earthly life, do you realize that you cannot take with you what you have accumulated? And that maybe everything is just hay straw and stubble, suitable for fire?

Or perhaps this doctrine teaches us to think about what happens after death? No, it does not; it does not prepare you for the most significant and most crucial examination without the appeal of your inner existence.

In his book "Think and Grow Rich," Napoleon Hill, in the section concerning the fundamental fears of man, states, "Death is like sleep, you don't have to be afraid of sleep."

It is not correct; death is not the end. Hebrews 9:27 says: How it is established that men die only once, after which comes judgment.

A being as deep as man, capable of loving, fighting, feeling deep emotions and feelings and learning the arts and science. Created perfect with eternity in the heart, it cannot end after the body's death.

There is only one way to true salvation, and as long as you have to find the true ikigai, this living and recent way is Jesus, put faith in him.

There are many religions and beliefs in the world, each one has its say, but here I am not presenting you with faith. Buddhism is the story of a man who became God. Christianity is the story of a God who became man. Buddhism says no harm; Christianity says love and does good. What remains of Buddha who died is still among us. Christ rose from the dead and is now at his father's right hand. Which law is superior? That of not doing evil? Or that of love?

When I pronounce the words religion and Christianity, I feel a particular revulsion at the meaning they have given to these terms as religious leaders; they arrogate to themselves the right to represent the Kingdom of God. Do they forget that the religious leaders of the time condemned Gesù to death? And that they were repeatedly harshly taken back by Jesus?

He defined them as "whitewashed tombs. Outwardly beautiful, pure and white, but inside full of death.

They talk about peace, but they make war, talk about love and hate. They speak of giving to others, but they live in the most unbridled riches. With their behavior, they prevent those in good faith from going directly to the source, placing themselves as a corrupt model to follow, obstructing the way to others.

Jesus did not live in luxurious houses; he did not wear pre-dressed clothes; he did not live in luxury; he did not need foreign symbols or signs. He put the needs of others before his own.

I went to the source and drank to the waters as well.

Gandhi said, "I like your Christ; I don't like your Christians. Your Christians are so different from your Christ."

You don't need any other mediator, and you don't need complications or men like you to free you. Basta believes in him and asks him to become your Lord and savior.

John 14:6 Jesus said to Him, "I am the way, the truth, and the life. No one comes to the Father except through me.

The Bible says," *"The word is near you, in your mouth, and your heart." This is the word of faith that we proclaim; because, if with your mouth you have confessed Jesus as Lord and believed with your heart that God raised him from the dead, you will be saved; with the heart, one feels* to obtain justice and with the mouth one makes a confession to be saved. "

You have to ask him to enter your heart and save you.

The following diagram **visually indicates what is exposed.**

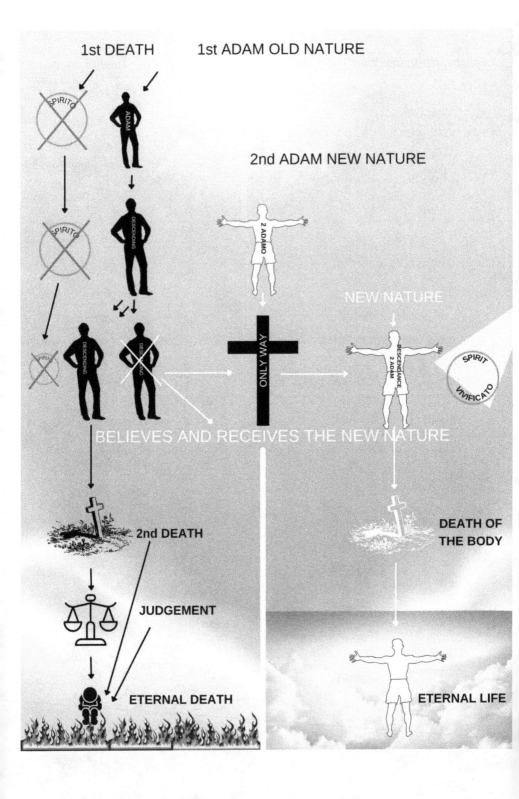

Putting into practice

We will see some phases of my life, during which we will see the concepts expressed so far applied in practical life. This part of the book is like an informal speech, which I do with my friends, with whom I share personal things, my intimate, not to get glory from them but to allow others to follow the same path that has given me results.

I often read beautiful books, but they stopped at the theoretical aspect. Now, I believe there is an abysmal distance between understanding something mechanically and mentally and experiencing it firsthand.

Every man is precious and vital, and every man has a calling is an essential purpose in his life. If we decide to live comfortably and not develop our ikigai, we may live far below our calling.

Accept mediocrity and strive for excellence, ask questions, push boundaries, seek answers, improve, learn, be stubborn but willing to listen, and live hungrily. Not the listener changes his life, but those who translate into action will be successful. Happy reading!!

The spark and the

fire

During the year 1992, many things have changed in my life. I had recently had a profound personal experience with Jesus. This choice and this experience will cost me a lot over time, but it will also give me much more than what I have lost. During this period, many friends have moved away from me. I had just turned 12 at the time, and I was a teenager. We know how vital the company he attends is for adolescence. Unfortunately, my father had lost his job, and we found ourselves in severe economic difficulty.

Let's go back a little in time to when it all began. I have always had an unconscious propensity for the search for God.

It was the summer of 1992, and with my friends, I was in the populous "Ferrubetina" district of Palmi, a small town in Calabria, where I was born and raised. After a few minutes, one of our friends left the house to join us. I had not seen him for a long time; he had always been an exceptionally polite and very respectful guy; in his way of doing things, something intrigued me.

During our conversations, with jokes and laughter, one of my friends offered to pick up a magazine so to speak, "uneducated" to watch together. My friend's reaction surprised me; he preferred to move away rather than glorify her. That gesture made me admire this boy, who behaved differently from the others, but I did not understand why. Later, I talked to Michele (fancy name), and he told me about a solid experience, which he had done shortly before in a youth camp. His way of speaking was utterly different from what I had heard so far about God. His experience was somehow alive, and he transmitted something active that drew me to this God.

His story was like a brush that painted a living picture in my heart, using bright colors, with bright and sparkling colors; a strong feeling of ardent love sprouted in me, which was kindled like a flame, for this wonderful God. I also wanted to be part of his army at any cost; it was what I wanted; I wanted nothing more than this.

I had seen God relegated to a simple religious function, but now he was presented to me differently.

I decided that what Michele had had had to be mine. Era what I was looking for, the answer to many doubts and inner conflicts.

The first test

I was just a little boy; in a contrary environment, I did not yet have a remarkable ability to resist the "bad weather of life."

In Calabria, there are many excellent and honest people. Many things make me proud of my land and my city Palmi (RC), such as the lush nature, the sea, the friendliness of many people who treat you like a family member even if they do not know you. My wonderful land is known and has become more so in recent years for many of its inhabitants; my wonderful land is known and has become more so for the mental backwardness of many of its inhabitants. For the solid criminal presence, the almost absence of the state, and for the nearly zero possibilities it offers to young people. To do something in Calabria, you have to fight ten times more than to do it elsewhere, and you will have to face a hostile environment.

I often felt discriminated against and sidelined during this time because I thought differently from others; it wasn't just my feeling. Still, I was an intelligent, friendly, and courteous guy.

When they learned of my choice, my relatives also thought of doing their part to "help" me change my mind, but it was not a simple idea; a fire had been lit in me, which, like a flame, could falter, but would not be extinguished. In particular, I remember my father took me to my paternal grandmother's house where all my uncles were gathered, I greeted them, but soon they would begin to do everything to discourage me from my faith. "Don't you care about the shame you make your father and mother have?" "Do you know that people make fun of you? "I was a kid, I felt like I was wrong, but I couldn't do anything about it because that was my desire, and I wouldn't give it up for anyone.

I still recur the question of one of my uncles. He had been a proud cop. Do you know that if you ask any general question about a carabinieri job, they will never accept you if they know of your faith? I replied to my uncle, aware that I could receive a loud slap from my father. I said: "If the carabinieri does not accept me for my faith, I do not want to be a cop." (*this discrimination does not happen, I esteem and am grateful to all the forces of the order for their contribution to security*).

Even though we had economic difficulties at that time, my father and mother gave us a lot of love and dignity. I do not tell these things to humiliate my parents, but to thank them for what they have done.

My parents always put my needs before theirs. I felt very loved. I remember that I had shoes that had opened downstairs and let water in those days. I tried not to make my parents notice and not to point it out to anyone. But I was freezing in a school, almost always skipping recess because I preferred not to ask my parents for money for a snack.

However, I did not seek anyone's compassion; I did not need it because I had found my life's purpose. There would be youth camping; it would cost 120,000 lire and last about ten days. The warning had been given a few months earlier so that we could save enough.

For me, it was impossible to think in the slightest about being able to participate in this event. In addition to not having the economic possibility, "my balance was zero," my parents were not happy with my choice. My father more than once tried to dissuade me; I do not blame him, one day he made me leave the house and told me not to return, he was not willing to do it, he left me on the stairs only for a few hours, he hoped that I would renounce my faith. But when I found myself alone, crying outside, I felt the presence of Jesus strongly. He was with me. His company was sweet, and nothing in the world, not even the best, could have been better than that experience.

He could understand how I felt because he had been rejected, and he was born in an animal stable. One day, my father was discouraged by my choice; that hurt me a lot; I didn't want to be selfish. He thought he had not been a good father, but it was not so; I had a great love for him, I embraced him, but he could not understand me.

My father has always loved me, but he could not understand that this was my life's purpose. He thought he wasn't a good father, but it was my personal choice.

After having my parents' disapproval this year, some of my childhood friends moved away from me.

One day, I met them, but they ran away as I tried to get closer. I understood that we would no longer be friends, but I didn't care; I wouldn't give up what was most important to me, anyone, and under any circumstances.

The youth camp was approaching with the summer, and finally, I received as a gift from my paternal grandmother 100,000 lire. I could have done many things with that money; I felt rich. I could have saved them for camping if my father had allowed me to go.

Or I could have bought myself something to eat for recreation for many days, or I could have bought myself new shoes.

Many of my schoolmates threw away food that was not to their liking; this created displeasure, as food may be wasted, for me, it was inconceivable; this would have meant more hunger at school, wet feet, and the end of my hopes of attending a youth camp.

When further communications were given about the campsite, it was displeasure. I would have liked more than anything else to go, but I could not. Nothing was in my favor; there was not the slightest chance to participate.

Despite the situation that should have discouraged me, I was not a depressed kid. Far from it, I was always joyful and smiling, and those who knew me knew that I had an innate propensity to joke.

Unfortunately, I had not been able to temporarily buy myself a Bible to be able to read it and understand something more; I limited myself to reading very short treatises, which were given to people.

Preparations for camping began, and communications multiplied. My new friends began to prepare what they needed in those days and exchanged advice on what to bring. The campsite was located in a beautiful destination in the Sila Woods. I was happy for them, but unfortunately, I would not have gone; therefore, I did not need to exchange councils.

The day of the camp arrived, but nothing had changed. I remember as if it were today that at 3 pm on a June afternoon, the bus full of young people would have left for a beautiful destination, in the middle of nature and the woods of Calabria.

Mi was about to spend most of my summer alone, without the possibility of even reading the Bible.

"Patience is like that," I said to myself. Anyway, around 2:20 pm, I went out to the veranda to stay a little alone. I was crying secretly, and I asked God how to ask a friend if it was possible to get me to go to that camp. My words were straightforward, and I did not use any particular or recited form of prayer. Only they came from the heart, with feeling and faith that God would hear.

At about 2:40 p.m., I heard the bell ring, my father replied. "Who is it? Yes, a moment I open." My father said kindly. "they want you." As I heard the gate close and someone down the stairs, I wondered who could ever be thinking of me at that moment. So, he went out on the stairs to meet him before my father saw him. When I recognized him I was left on ice, he was the father of one of my new friends, and he was coming to ask me to go to the campsite. Quietly I told him, "thank you, but I can't come; it is better not to say anything to my father because I believe he will react very badly."

He did not care what I had just told him, and with a smile, he told me, "be quiet"; come, could that man have such absolute calm. I was very agitated.

What my eyes saw a few moments later has no possible explanation. I mention my father and our difficult moment; I would never have asked for such a sacrifice.

Contrary to what I expected, my father was very kind; I could not believe my eyes. Until that moment, I had been terrified of it. Every time I did something "for God," I risked receiving severe punishment.

Without giving me any rational explanation, I found myself preparing my clothes to leave from there in a few minutes with amazement.

My father, he slept me; I hugged him, kissed him and went down with my friend's father.

To avoid offending my father, I did not bring up the subject in front of him but told my friend's father when I was away. "I can't afford to come."

I was already thinking about what to say when he saw me come back not to hurt him.

I would have expected him to tell me something like, "ah, I'm sorry, it will be for next time." Instead, he kept telling me, "don't worry." But I was worried I would have made a wrong impression.

When I got to the bus, I told the manager with a thread of voice I didn't have the money to pay. I thought it would have been harder for me to get to my destination and then have to find a way home, so I found the courage to say it right away. But he replied, "Don't worry, someone didn't want to come, and you took his place."

Someone had pronounced it last minute because he did not want to go there. He did not have a burning desire. One could not wish to go to this camp of young people, where I could meet many of my peers, have fun, make friends, and meet God more profoundly.

Arriving at the camp, I met many young people who had had the same experience as me; now, we had a lot in common, and it was simply wonderful to see that these guys managed to be joyful, playful, and full of life despite leading a life close to God.

I had always thought that being religious meant living a sacrificed and joyless life. That it was necessary to retire to read and meditate away from everyone and everything, closed in some boring monastery. That life wasn't for me.

But these young people, full of joy and vitality, were showing me the opposite, it was possible to have fun and have friends, to lead a happy and entire life even with simple things, even if they were close to God. They didn't need to say bad words or smoke, and they didn't need to be religious wands. Before, a guy who smoked was free to do what he wanted, but my concept changed. A boy who smoked was a slave to that thing. These young people were free, and they did not need these things.

I was repaid abundantly for lost friendships, taunts, and discrimination in that camp. There was a different friendship between these guys and me, more profound and sincere. That summer was the happiest summer of my life, nothing I had done before was comparable, and I did not need entertainment because I led the whole life and had found the purpose of existence.

That year, you learned that when you give something to God ultimately, even if it is defective, God repays you with something significantly better. I also knew that you could get it when you have a burning desire for something. I didn't need to read a manual or read it somewhere; I experimented with it.

Always refusing to abandon it to please my friends, gain employment, or be accepted. I had given him, without knowing it, my future and my finances. Good gave me back much more than what I had given before.

During this time, I had the opportunity to establish friendships that were nothing short of fraternal, a quality that was unimaginable before.

We loved God, yes, but at the same time, we were teenagers, and now and then, we combined some jokes. I remember one evening after dinner, while we spent the evening in joy with other young people, a little boy who would become a great friend of mine, coming out of a door where there was a room, a wedding dinner had just ended. His name was Gianmarco (fancy name)." With an amused air, I asked him, "but what are you combining." I knew that if he was in the middle, fun was guaranteed. And he, with a sly smile, replied.

"There was a wedding, and some intact sweets were leftover; the waiters said I could take them. They would have been lost otherwise, so I quietly entered the room, closed the door, and began to eat what we could.

The quantities of food at the campsite were not very abundant, so we were occasionally hungry. But I didn't complain about the food; I was grateful to have it. Gratitude to God opens the doors for a happy and long life; even during difficulties, you can have joy.

I appreciated Gianmarco because he was unconventional, very lovely, and often invented some of his "strategies" to do something. He was very polite; all the boys were; Gianmarco had a great love for God, which made us have a lot in common.

The principles set out

I hope to have succeeded in this story to make you grasp the aspects expressed in a theoretical way used in real life. I trust you could learn the flow, resilience, life purpose, and divine response when we get serious.

Constance resilience

Whatever you decide to do, whatever path you choose to take, you will be tried at some point.

We do not get to the next step if a test does not come first, and so in the Old Testament, it is so for each of us. The test serves for a threefold reason.

1. We find our faith constancy, resilience, and ardent desire.
2. The creator tries to see if we are ready to receive more.
3. We want to show the material, spiritual world what our direction is.

When we embark on something new that excites us in the early stages, we receive strength and stimulation from what we can call "the first love." The first love is a solid feeling, capable of shaking mountains, and it is that feeling that allows a lover to travel miles and miles to see his beloved. However, this fantastic condition is bound to diminish over time; this is the stage when many marriages fail; the first love can hide flaws. At this stage, we are so in love that everything is perfect. This love can be directed towards a person but also other material things. The quality of the love we have for our girlfriend or wife determines the stability of our marital future.

When the infatuation ends, we see flaws; what was perfect is now annoying. If we do not have developed true love in this new phase, that is, that which gives and covers up the mistakes, we will live our marriage badly. Man's love is selfish, "I love you because you are beautiful and because I feel good near you." The center of love is not the other person but me that receives well at that moment. Divine love is of a different quality; he loves us with a perfect love with all our faults, so much so that he gave his life for us, so we must love. We often hear you say; I don't love you anymore.

Returning to our lives, this is the stage in which we should develop resilience and constancy. Chi relies on the only love is, known as infatuation. At some point, he stops feeling this feeling, and its disappearance will also end the determination.

Over the years, I have met many people, paraphrasing the life of faith with athletic life. These people looked like born athletes; it was fantastic to see that they had made incredible progress in a short time, so much so that they seemed favored to win the Olympics. Unfortunately, however, our life is more like a marathon than a sprint of 100 meters, and time tests everyone's faith. Many of these people are no longer traceable; they stopped from the race.

When feelings begin to blow against you, you will need more equipment. It is tough to learn to separate one's path from one's feelings; it is difficult not to be conditioned by them.

But if you want to reach your ikigai, you will have to learn to do without feelings. At this point, you will need:

Faith creates a vision; When you have faith in something, you imagine it, you imagine yourself doing that something, and you dream of reaching a goal. This is the vision that only you can have and

112

understand; remember not to seek approval from others because they may not understand your vision. A surfer rode a strange wave; according to the spectators in the stands, that man was considered a madman, no one would have regarded as the sea a safe place, except for one person, the person who had the faith and vision.

But often, others watch from the stands from a safe place; 99.99% of people are there. They seem to tell you insistently, get out of there, you will get hurt; you do not see that it is crazy anyone with a shred of common sense would do what you do.

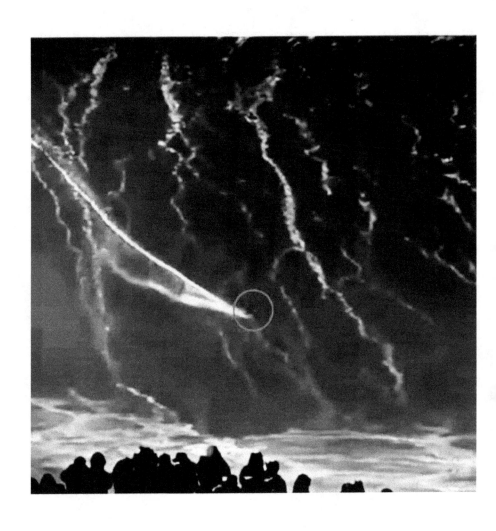

On the other hand, what they shout from the stands is true, it is true for them. They would die instead of the surfer because they do not have faith, constancy, tenacity, and preparation. I point out that this was true for everyone except one in the middle of the wave. Faith is inextricably linked to action; if there is no action, faith is dead; when activity ceases, faith ceases. You believe what you're doing, and you don't think what you think is right.

If you want to excel, you have to live with disapproval. Today's society has thought patterns that are not easy to escape.

The collective exerts a very high psychological pressure, and almost impossible to get rid of it, and the first love will end at some point. If you do something, you are not to some extent disapproved, always talking about lawful and pure things; you can consider it as an indication that something is wrong. If you overcome the fence of society, they will do everything to get you back inside; many reactions will also be violent and continuous; this will happen especially with people very close to you.

Here is because you will need resilience and constancy. Resilience is a muscle that a man develops every time he faces adversity and refuses to give in. Resilience is one of the essential ingredients without which you will not be able to achieve results, and when the feeling of first love fades, so will the results.

It should also be noted that the surfer had to do a complex preparation before reaching that level and being able to ride that wave. Thinking of achieving a goal without adequate preparation is not faith but presumption.

Before this emblematic image where the surfer defies the laws of nature, resilience had made resilience his companion. I imagine all the falls, the broken boards, the money spent, and probably sometimes he will have even hurt himself and risked drowning. But his great desire fueled his resilience to reach the right level at the right time. In addition to the resistance, he had to have constancy. Constancy has to do with gait and rhythm; we often hear phrases in sport such as: "athletes are keeping a steady pace." A constant pace allows you to dose the energies to be able to get to the bottom, and it is known that even a car that travels on the highway at a constant speed consumes less.

An athlete who does not keep a constant pace according to his speed but adapts to the rate of others without adequate preparation most likely will not see the finish line. Constancy also allows us to know ourselves and our limits to overcome them. Constancy shapes our body and spirit, giving us the characteristics we need to achieve the goal. It takes endurance for the surfer to get out of bed on cold and rainy days to train when no one sees him. But all his constancy, faith, determination, and concentration are enjoyed harmoniously on the day of his performance.

My ikigai at work

Many Years after my first experience, I have gone through the work phases that I want to describe. I had already been in the military, and I had always worked to help the domestic economy. During these times, I received many things using faith, but now I will focus on a later time frame. During 2005, I worked as an employee at a shipyard; this entrance was significant for my economic dependence. I relentlessly pursued the goal of improving my working life and knew that to achieve a result that others had not completed, I had to act differently from what they did.

I have always acted by trying to listen to my inner voice, the voice with which God speaks to us. Sometimes this voice manifests itself through peace; other times, you do not feel comfortable doing a sure thing, while other times, still, it can be audible. However, when you open yourself to the guide, god somehow makes you understand what is good for you. When I have not heard this voice, I have always had negative experiences. My advice is if you want the best for your life, ask God. And he is not like a master father ready with a stick, but he will answer you. If you have never tried to do it, I challenge you to try genuinely. Another piece of advice I can give you is to have a sentimentally neutral attitude towards the situation you need confirmation from above. God does not cry out, Does not interfere in our choices; he respects our free will. Since the divine response, many times can be similar to a feeling, if we do not place ourselves in a neutral situation, being willing to give up that thing, we will not be able to listen to the divine voice, and we will be convinced that that is the right way. So before we give free rein to our feelings, let us place ourselves for a period in a state of neutrality until we have an answer.

At that time, I was working in this shipyard, and it was not my highest aspiration; it still gave me economic security and had entered my comfort zone. I was used to that job, I had reached certain financial independence, and what I was doing was good.

Purtroppo, but the good and enemy of the best, I could have settled in that lukewarm and accommodating situation, but it was not for me. At that moment, I felt divine approval for that work, and honestly, there was no point in changing. Until I slowly began to have a certain restlessness during my career, I did not feel satisfied. I knew it was no longer my place. Perciò decided to fire me and stand still for a while to wait for other instructions. At that time, I had met that girl who would become my wife in the future. Being from another region, we could not see each other very often; my in-laws, who love me so much, would have been pleased to see me more often, given that there was the possibility of hosting me in the apartment below. It was not conceivable to relax, and I would have been ashamed to be hosted at their expense.

When my father-in-law had been running an insurance company for years, he would have been happy to fit me into his office. More their house was structured so that the children could have an independent dwelling in the same building.

118

But my inner voice insistently told me that I should stay where I was. I might have seemed unsense to reject everything for nothing. At that time, I had no job prospects, I didn't own a house, and I didn't have specific training. All I could offer was uncertainty.

All I had was my faith that God would change things and Bless me.

Perci that summer, I waited because I knew my cousin was looking for someone to work in his car practice agency; at the time, the guy who worked with him had resigned; if I hadn't been free from my job, I would not have been able to take advantage of this opportunity. My father then asked my uncle to let me work. My uncle, whom I adore, responded negatively because the experience was required, and according to him, I would not have been able to manage the sector's most demanding client.

Later, they agreed that my father, who had previously worked in that office for some time, would support me for free until I could be a valuable helper. So time passed, and I learned the job. I had decided after praying that that agency of car practices should become mine; I felt the divine approval, but I had no means to do it. Moreover, my uncle and my cousin had no intention of giving it up.

Perciò I began to make it an object of continuous prayer with faith, I also bought a miniature model of a motorcycle, and I said this I will put it in my agency when it was not mine yet in reality.

I was moved by faith, asking the God of the invisible to move the mountains in my favor. It was a crazy undertaking, and only with a vision of faith could I get a response. Faith creates an image; our mind imagines the materialization of the divine response; this is how faith makes a vision. The answer often happens just like you imagine. Other times it happens in different ways and at different times. With

119

experience, I have learned that it is not advisable to force the hand by doing one's own thing but that the answer will come in due course. In the meantime, we must take actions that go in that direction and continue to ask God with faith and gratitude.

I can guarantee you that if you decide to rely on him, you will not be disappointed; this thing is more true than the sun that rises in the morning.

Stop and be grateful

During these periods, I had fallen, and many times I felt defeated and discouraged; I found an excellent medicine in gratitude to God. When we get depressed, we often have a limited vision. We are probably already seeing a negative future, stopping and starting to focus on everything that, by grace and divine goodness, we have is a formidable cure. When I felt futureless and defeated, I began to thank God for waking up that day, for having the ability to breathe, to walk, to sleep, so that I could think; then, I thanked God for the things I didn't like because they could have been much worse. There was always a way to be grateful. Gratitude and thanksgiving have often taken me out of health and work conditions. Let's think about it; we can always be grateful. Maybe you could reply, if only you knew my condition, there would be nothing to be grateful for; this is not true. It is a deception; every human being passes through trials. There was a period in my life that I will not dwell much on when I had great difficulty in health; I believed that my life would not last long, I had trouble even walking, but this did not prevent me from being grateful. At times I was overwhelmed by discouragement, but who knows me knows that at that moment, I sought God's help more and regularly spent time thanking him. Suffering can teach us something. What I am telling you was not theoretical for me; for this reason, I tell you that you can rebuild your life now, no matter how low you feel or what happens, you can do it now by grace.

Every promise has it's yes and amen

After more than a year of continuous prayer and faith, the conditions for buying the agency are miraculously being realized. My father had tried for years to sell land and would have helped me with a portion of the proceeds, but he had failed.

I reiterate that when I began to ask God for this, there was no possibility of realization. Perciò, in the end, with the help of my father, who I will never thank enough, I managed to find an agreement for the acquisition. I gave the deposit to my uncle, and everything seemed to have ended in the best way. Just when the victory of faith and constancy had already manifested itself, my uncle thought again, returned the deposit to me, and put my cousin to work, then I was a bit disappointed, but I immediately started looking for another job. A few more months passed, and my uncle again decided to sell the agency. I didn't want to be disappointed again, so I bought the agency's stock on the advice of another uncle.

The agency came from a moment of decay due to these continuous shocks; from when I took over the business to when I closed it, I always recorded growth in work and the number of customers. Di this was aware everyone in my sector, and I had become the reference point for many operators in the industry. I worked full time from 400 cases managed the first year to nearly 4,000 the last year. Except for one year, I've seen a steady increase in customers.

I have always tried to give my best in terms of professionalism and speed.

The creative mind

I said that you have to have a creative mind rather than a competitive mind. What do I mean by this is that it is much better to create something different than compete.

I will try to give you an example of how I have applied it to my work. I often analyzed my business and thought about how I could improve it by experimenting with new things.

An automotive consulting firm comes into play when two parties, buyer and seller of any motor vehicle, meet and conclude the negotiation. They choose where to complete the transfer of ownership; clients could have chosen both other agencies and me; my strategy was to get involved before there was the choice of a consulting firm, and that is to help the client sell his car. I have founded an agency to mediate car sales between private individuals. If what allowed me to anticipate my competition, I came into play before buyer-seller met. At that point, I increased my range of services, such as offering a guarantee policy between individuals or the possibility of carrying out a financing practice. I also used software designed ad hoc that allowed me to multi-post sales ads. In addition, the ads were placed in a local newspaper in the sector, and for this premium service, who decided to put his machine for sale had to pay me a small advance, this allowed me to have free advertising. In addition to this, I also carried out real marketing techniques that I am not going to list because we will dwell too long. I recently met with a large company that provides software for our sector. I had presented the idea that they had welcomed positively and with whom I could collaborate shortly to develop a service to offer to other agencies.

I will not dwell on the many activities and improvements that I have developed in my consulting firm, but this is to tell you how much more profitable it is to use **a creative and non-competitive mind. When you compete, you** compete on the price; when you create something new, you say the conditions.

However, our activity must always pass through the divine response. After over a decade in which I had many job satisfactions and divine abundance, I decided to listen to my inner voice and, after asking God to change activities. The consulting firm carries many responsibilities and occupies most of the day. I felt the need to have more space and free time, it was my desire, and I was convinced that God would help me. When we don't like something, we complain and tend to externalize the causes of our dissatisfaction. If you want to find your ikigai, you have to take responsibility for your **situation.**

- If only I had had more consideration;
- If only I had been more paid;
- If only life had been less unjust.

Complaining does not bring any results, and it only leads to wasting energy that you could use better. I often complained in some situations, but then I realized that I was responsible. I have **Replaced the "I want to be paid more" with the "I have to be worth more."** If they pay me little, I will probably do a job that does not require a great specialization; specialization is the key to happy working life. Please pay attention to it; the more specialized a doctor is, the more we have to pay him and dictates his conditions

Significant changes always require a lot of energy. During the stages of development, children will often have a fever and will have to go through pain, but this is necessary for there to be development; we can not live like dwarfs. Usually, when significant changes happen in my life, I see this process triggered in me:

1. I start to feel dissatisfied with what I am doing; I speak in terms of work or activity. Most people stop and use the narcotic of complaint and apology; they will never embark on the journey. We might think, *"What's the use of striving, so nothing will ever change? It takes luck, I'll go for a coffee with my friends, and I'll get distracted so as not to think".* You must listen to your **dissatisfaction, not indulge or narcotize it.**

2. I ask God daily to help me choose what is best for me. More miserly, you will need to know that he is guiding you like a reliable GPS, will be your guide, and will avoid turning around when you have no landmarks.

3. Dissatisfaction increases, but at the same time, I begin to look for alternatives on an ongoing basis. It is essential to spend enough time at this stage. It is like when the flour rises, which needs the correct times and the proper doses.

4. Always maintaining a neutral attitude and openness to the divine voice, I begin to devote some time to the new activity that I have found to do. Remember that we talked about price? When I started my new self-publishing business, I had to find the time to do this thing that I was passionate about; I was constantly working from 7 pm after a busy working day when I closed until one to two in the morning. Every day I repeated, I

had to succeed, failure was not contemplated, I could have made mistakes 1000 times, and 1000 times I would have started from scratch. I had to have no free time for a long time. That year I ultimately gave up taking a vacation, and I spent my summer without going to the beach, closed inside the consulting firm to work on the new skills I needed. Divine guidance, faith, ardent desire, constancy, and action were my fellow workers. You decide that no fall will do it for you; you can get up again. **You have to keep your mind focused long enough on what you want to do for it to acquire it. Defeat should not be taken seriously as part of the process, and it must exist.** A phrase that I continuously repeated to myself and gave me a great boost was, "if someone has *excellent results in this activity, then I can have them too." 1000 and 1000 people still will be ready to share their negative experiences with you, experiences undoubtedly real as accurate* as their faith in this failure. You point your eyes up and see who does better than you. Always observe and ask yourself many questions; observation, humility, and questions will take you from the bottom up; you always start from the bottom. "*Why is this person paid more than me? what does it do differently from what I do?* "Without jealousy, the jealous will not succeed, but go with your best and observe them.

5. It was not a random response to my actions but a precise response to my efforts. It was not a spontaneous response to my actions but an accurate response. At this stage is the time when is learning; your mind will try to sabotage you and make you go back. Remember that you will be tested for each person and what will try to sabotage your decision. There is a middle ground between the old and the new activity; that land is called

a desert. Io I crossed it, the desert happens when you can no longer go back to what you did before, and when what you will have to do has not yet given you any fruit. Many carcasses of dreams and good intentions lie permanently in the desert, this is the time when feelings of nostalgia appear, and you wonder but what have I done? But if you do not pass by there you will not be able to go on, better to die fighting than to live as a sheep.

This is what you need faith for, to see the answer that you do not yet see, the constancy not to decrease your gait, if you do not keep a certain step it will not overcome the desert. The ardent desire that must be renewed continuously because it burns in your life, And the action without which faith is dead

End

A I still have a lot of things to write, but I think it's right to offer you a balanced reading. If these concepts are new to you, you have a lot to digest. You may have noticed that I wanted you to see these principles in action in a book that is not very technical but more practical. I advise you to read it and reread it many times because often you will find concepts that will be very important only in the future for your success. Some principles we do not assimilate until we are in a favorable condition; many things exposed will have more value for you at other stages of your life.

I hope you have been able to find this valuable text for your life and that you can make the best of it. If you were created wonderfully and uniquely, there is no other particular person like you, nor will he ever exist. Be aware of your worth, and remember that God has loved you so much so that you may have peace and joy.

I want to thank you again for the choice of this humble literary work; if you're going to stay in touch with me and want to receive updates on my activities, you can write to me at the email: gaecel.gf@gmail.com

I would be grateful if you would share your experience with other readers by posting a short review. I hope to be able to read your comment soon. I greet you warmly!!

CLICK. FROM KINDLE OR SCAN THE QR-CODE!!

Gaetano Fortugno

To show you my gratitude, I want to GIVE YOU THIS VERY USEFUL BOOK. Thank you!!

CLICK. From kindle or scan the QR-Code!!

Here is the answer to the 9-point game:

If you have succeeded, congratulations for finding the answer; you are undoubtedly an excellent problem solver! If you have not succeeded, do not give up; there are only a few people who can solve this game.

The game serves to think outside the box. You couldn't solve this problem because you saw it as a square and reasoned to solve a square.

This implies that we must not allow ourselves to be conditioned by the limits of the grid. In reality, the lines that need to be drawn must extend beyond these limits.

When you start to think differently from others, you will find different solutions. Tell God to influence your life. We are influenced by society and rules more than we imagine. Often we think that there is no solution to a situation, everyone may believe that it is so, without solution, but just think outside the square, the vast majority of people live inside a square. By reversing like this, with a renewed mind, I was able to solve many problems that I thought were insurmountable.

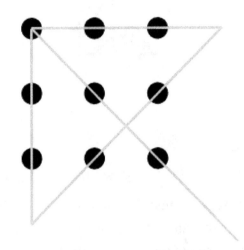